Intermittent Fasting 16/8

*What is Intermittent Fasting?
Discover the Ultimate 16/8 Diet
Plan to Lose Weight and Recover
Your Energy*

Linden Roderick

Table of Contents

Introduction: How to Lose Weight

Do you want to lose weight permanently? Or have you tried to lose weight only to regain most of it back in a few months or years? If so, you'll find this book extremely useful because it shows you how to lose weight permanently in a natural way. But before I tell you how this book will help you, let me tell you an astonishing story.

The Story of the Biggest Loser

In 2016, researchers wanted to find out if "The Biggest Loser" participants went on to experience metabolic adaptation years after the 30-week competition. Not only that, they were also curious if the degree of metabolic adaptation was related to weight regain. These experts believed metabolism decreased as the body composition changed during weight loss. Perhaps you are wondering what we mean by metabolic adaptation. Not to worry.

Metabolic adaptation simply means the body's response to fight back against attempts to lose weight. This means that if you try to lose weight, the body reacts to counter this by adjusting the chemistry in the body to maintain or regain the weight.

What was "The Biggest Loser" competition? It was an American reality show broadcast on NBC from 2004 to 2016. The competition dangled a carrot to be obtained by the participant who lost the biggest percentage of weight during the 30-week period. Participants who were overweight or obese, were subjected to a calorie-restricted diet plus an intensive, supervised training regime.

Researchers recruited 14 of the 16 participants to investigate their theories on metabolic adaptation. What they did was measure a number of variables including resting metabolic rate (RMR) and body composition measures such as insulin, leptin, insulin resistance, fats, and adiponectin. The resting metabolic rate was performed after the former contestants fasted overnight for 12 hours.

This study, performed six years after the end of the competition, got the green light from the Institutional Review Board of the National Institute of Diabetes and Digestive and Kidney Disease to go ahead.

Before the participants entered the competition, their overall baseline weight was 148,9kg (328.3 lbs.). At the end of the competition, this cohort had lost an average of 58.3kg (128.5 lbs.), which means the participants weighed 90.6kg (199.7 lbs.) at the close of the competition.

What Were the Results?

Our savvy experts were stunned by what they discovered. For example, 13 of the 14 recruits had gained back some of the weight they had lost during the popular TV series. This means only one participant who lost weight managed to keep it off permanently. But why? We'll come back to this question later. Let's first continue looking at the results of this study. Here's a table summarizing the results:

	Baseline	End of competition at 30 weeks	Follow-up at 6 years	Baseline vs. 30 weeks	Baseline vs. 6 years	30 weeks vs. 6 years
Age (years)	34.9 ± 10.3	35.4 ± 10.3	41.3 ± 10.3	<0.0001	<0.0001	<0.0001
Weight (kg)	148.9 ± 40.5	90.6 ± 24.5	131.6 ± 45.3	<0.0001	0.0294	0.0002
BMI (kg/m^2)	49.5 ± 10.1	30.2 ± 6.7	43.8 ± 13.4	<0.0001	0.0243	0.0002
% Body fat	49.3 ± 5.2	28.1 ± 8.9	44.7 ± 10	<0.0001	0.0894	0.0003
FM (kg)	73.4 ± 22.6	26.2 ± 13.6	61.4 ± 30	<0.0001	0.0448	0.0001
FFM (kg)	75.5 ± 21.1	64.4 ± 15.5	70.2 ± 18.3	<0.0001	0.0354	0.0101
RQ	0.77 ± 0.05	0.75 ± 0.03	0.81 ± 0.02	0.272	0.0312	<0.0001
RMR measured (kcal/d)	$2,607 \pm 649$	$1,996 \pm 358$	$1,903 \pm 466$	0.0004	<0.0001	0.3481
RMR predicted (kcal/d)	$2,577 \pm 574$	$2,272 \pm 435$	$2,403 \pm 507$	<0.0001	0.0058	0.0168
Metabolic adaptation (kcal/d)	29 ± 206	-275 ± 207	-499 ± 207	0.0061	<0.0001	0.0075
TEE (kcal/d)	$3,804 \pm 926$	$3,002 \pm 573$	$3,429 \pm 581$	0.0014	0.0189	0.0034
Physical activity (kcal/kg/d)	5.6 ± 1.8	10.0 ± 4.6	10.1 ± 4.0	0.0027	0.001	0.8219

Figure 1: Results of a followup study of The Biggest Loser competition

As you can see, six years after the end of the competition, the participants continued to burn fewer calories than at the beginning. There was a small difference between resting metabolic rate at the end of the competition and at followup time. Now, because our participants regained weight, we would expect the metabolic rate to climb up. But this data suggests otherwise. From this data, we can postulate that the lifestyle of the participants may have changed after the competition, including what they ate and how they trained. This means they may have burnt fewer calories than they consumed, forcing the body to store some fuel as fat.

Let's find out what happened with body composition measurements. Here's a table summarizing those results:

	Baseline	End of competition at 30 weeks	Follow-up at 6 years	P Baseline vs. 30 weeks	Baseline vs. 6 years	30 weeks vs. 6 years
Glucose (mg/dL)	95.7 ± 16.3	70.2 ± 21.9	104.9 ± 48.7	0.0042	0.4759	0.0264
Insulin (µU/mL)	10.4 ± 8.5	3.9 ± 1.9	12.1 ± 7.5	0.0126	0.3204	0.0013
C-peptide (ng/mL)	3 ± 1.4	1.3 ± 0.9	2.7 ± 1.1	0.0019	0.4241	0.0016
HOMA-IR	2.5 ± 2.2	0.7 ± 0.4	3.6 ± 4.6	0.0134	0.1892	0.0431
TG (mg/dL)	126.5 ± 76.3	57.4 ± 22.3	92.9 ± 43.9	0.0019	0.053	0.0082
Cholesterol (mg/dL)	174 ± 41.2	192.4 ± 52.6	180.9 ± 45.9	0.2115	0.5945	0.3549
LDL (mg/dL)	105 ± 30	126 ± 46	108 ± 35	0.132	0.8343	0.1083
HDL (mg/dL)	42.5 ± 17.6	54.6 ± 14.9	54.5 ± 21.2	0.0036	0.001	0.9751
Adiponectin (mg/mL)	2.46 ± 1.28	4.69 ± 2.05	7.29 ± 4.71	0.0003	0.0025	0.0164
T3 (ng/dL)	9.42 ± 2.78	5.31 ± 1.45	11.15 ± 1.81	0.0006	0.0623	<0.0001
T4 (µg/dL)	7.3 ± 1.58	6.95 ± 1.43	6.18 ± 1.12	0.3814	0.0486	0.0828
TSH (µIU/mL)	1.52 ± 1.26	1.42 ± 0.73	1.93 ± 0.9	0.7175	0.1933	0.0641
Leptin (ng/mL)	41.14 ± 16.91	2.56 ± 2.19	27.68 ± 17.48	<0.0001	0.013	0.0001

Figure 2: Body composition results of The Biggest Loser competitors

It is evident that leptin, the hunger hormone, increased between the end of competition and at followup. It isn't surprising that the majority of the participants regained some of the lost weight. They probably could not resist the urge to eat tasty dishes and snacks such as chocolate and pizza. Just look at the insulin level. At the followup time, it had gone even higher than at the start of the competition. And insulin plays a role in the regulation of glucose in the bloodstream.

Despite the metabolic adaptation coming out as expected, the astonishing finding is that five of the participants at followup were within 1% of their weight at the start of the competition. We must wonder why, even after such a rigorous program, did some participants regain so much weight.

You see, losing weight should be seen as a process of adjusting your lifestyle. Once you adopt a healthy lifestyle, you never should have to worry about regaining weight after losing some. This is because the weight you lose would simply be a result of lifestyle changes. The best part is that a lifestyle change tends to follow the natural way change in general takes place. Rapid weight loss, like in "The Biggest Loser" competition, rarely helps build new sustainable habits. This is where intermittent fasting 16/8 and this book come in.

Intermittent fasting is not a fad. Intermittent fasting is a way of life that aligns very well with how the human body already functions. Unfortunately, in this civilized world, our bodies have forgotten their natural way of functioning. What is required is to reset the body and keep it that way -- and that process is easy with intermittent fasting 16/8.

Take Jannie's story of how she used intermittent fasting 16/8 to shed 65 pounds. Jannie tipped the scale at 337 lbs. One day, she sat on her bed watching her fast asleep 3-year-old daughter. Right at that moment, she felt fear hit her hard. She thought she wouldn't see the following day in her life -- that she would die. Why? You see, this beautiful African American girl felt pain and had breathing difficulties while asleep at night. On that night, watching her growing daughter sleeping, she made a life-changing decision. She fixed her mind upon seeing her daughter grow up with a mother.

That's when she decided to begin intermittent fasting 16/8. She says it was hard at first, but patiently persisted. Later, she added mild daily training by simply walking 15 minutes on a treadmill. Fast-forward 7 months, she had lost 65 pounds.

You see, to lose weight, all you have to do is burn more calories than you are consuming on a daily basis. If you do that over a period of time, the body begins to burn body fat as it adjusts the metabolic rate. It is the intention of this book to show you how to burn your body fat via intermittent fasting 16/8. But before you begin with the actual fasting process, there are certain foundational elements that must be in place for you to lose weight permanently. As the ancient masters said, "know thyself and you shall know the gods." It is vital you know how your body works to be able to shed body weight safely and keep it off.

That's why this book begins by discussing a key subject called digestion. In this chapter, we begin by discussing hunger, what it is, and what causes it. This understanding will help you manage any hunger that occurs during fasting. Immediately thereafter, we dive into the path that food takes until it is turned into nutrients and excreted waste. We begin with what happens to food in your mouth, esophagus, stomach, small intestine and the large intestine. Not only that, there are specific hormones that play a significant role in effective digestion.

Once we finish discussing digestion, we'll go on to talk about the science of intermittent fasting in chapter 2. Here, we will define what fasting and intermittent fasting are and the benefits thereof. Most importantly, we delve into the subject of ketosis, what it is and how our bodies enter into this state. We also talk about a subject that concerns diabetics who may want to lose weight through intermittent fasting called ketoacidosis. We explain what it means and what its impact on the body could be.

You see, most of us try to use willpower to effect sustainable weight loss. Unfortunately, the majority after successful weight loss, quickly regain their weight. And we are quick to blame the birth of our kids, hunger, cravings, and countless other reasons for putting on massive pounds again. Luckily, science has discovered that there's a lawbreaker most of us don't know about that is at fault. But everyone of us can manage this lawbreaker.

Chapter 3 goes into detail how this lawbreaker works and how we can get it to work for us, instead of against us. Here, we seek the assistance of experts to get guidance on what controls our behavior. Weight gain is a result of doing things in a certain way. If we understand what causes us to do the things that lead to weight gain, we can intelligently make informed choices supported by the natural workings of our bodies.

Chapter 4 discusses a concept most diet programs fail to recognize. There is a general belief that we all respond the same way to available diets. Most western governments have produced nutritional guidelines that assume people's bodies respond the same way to eating the same type of food. A recent research report revealed shocking information that stunned even the researchers on how people respond to meals. You see, blood glucose levels play a significant role in fat build-up in the body. So, controlling glucose levels is essential. This chapter will discuss research into this glucose behavior in different people. Researchers were surprised by the results as much as I was, and I suspect you will be amazed as well.

Chapter 5 explains how to get started with intermittent fasting 16/8. It is vital to check with your physician before adopting any fasting regime. Most importantly, you need to get measurements such as blood glucose, weight, and heart rate done to use as your baseline. We also give you a guiding schedule to safely and effectively begin your weight loss fasting lifestyle. This chapter further discusses why it's essential to start with a bigger eating period and progressively make small adjustments on a day-by-day basis until you hit your targeted fasting program of 16/8. Once you get started with intermittent fasting 16/8, you'll want to know what kind of foods facilitate weight loss with fasting. Most importantly, not everyone should undertake fasting, and we reveal what type of people in this chapter.

Chapter 6 delves into the kinds of foods that are suitable for our bodies. There are some food items that do not support weight loss. Yes, with intermittent fasting you may eat any food you like during the feeding cycle. However, there are certain kinds of food that are detrimental to our bodies and health, and you must know about them. Best of all, we'll talk about the importance of testing various foods because as chapter 4 shows, the same food may not have the same effect on everyone. For example, a piece of bread may increase glucose levels in the bloodstream of one person, and have no effect on another.

It is important to know before you start with intermittent fasting 16/8 that there are other benefits that you would never have thought about. It is the intention of chapter 7 to give the details of these benefits. The human body is a complex combination of systems such as the digestive system, reproductive system, endocrine system, and so on. A change in one system tends to affect other systems, and ultimately the body. In fact, for weight loss to occur, there must be a change in the endocrine system, which then influences the digestive system, and finally, weight loss. This chapter will discuss seven other benefits that accrue due to successful implementation of intermittent fasting 16:8.

Chapter 8 goes into detail about concerns intermittent fasters may have. Some fasters have raised a concern that they don't seem to be losing weight. We dive deep into eight possible reasons for this and also provide ways to overcome those challenges. Other concerns discussed include whether intermittent fasting causes insomnia, gastritis, headaches, diarrhea, and a few others.

Lastly, we end the book with a concluding chapter for you to use as a reference source whenever you need a quick reminder of key ideas from the book. Perhaps this chapter is ideal to read immediately after this introduction to have a helicopter view of the main ideas covered in the book. So, if indeed losing weight is important to you, you hold in your hands a practical guide on how to do so safely and effectively.

Go ahead and enjoy reading and implementing the ideas we suggest to lose weight permanently and gain more energy than you've ever done before.

Chapter 1: Digestion 101 - A Quick Lesson on How Your Body Turns Food into Energy and Fat

Common sense says people should eat food to satisfy hunger. Just look at what people around you do. Do they eat to simply satisfy hunger? Certainly not. Today, we eat food not just to satisfy hunger, but to avoid boredom and to satisfy our huge appetites. It is this latter kind of eating that causes many of us to develop massive waistlines, excessive belly fat and concerning health issues. Of these diseases, perhaps obesity, cardiovascular diseases, diabetes, and liver diseases are the most worrisome. That's partly why we may choose to alter our diets.

The success of any effort to lose weight, including intermittent fasting 16/8, depends on the type of knowledge we have and our willingness to apply it. Applying that knowledge depends very much on having the right information for the purpose at hand. Hence, we need to understand what the body does with the food that we eat. In this chapter, we'll cover the full path that food takes from mouth right through to excretion (removal of waste from the large intestine). In addition, we'll discuss the processes that take place in each of the main organs of digestion. But first, let us talk about hunger.

What is Hunger and What Causes It?

In simple language, hunger is the body's way of telling us that the body needs to refuel to continue to function normally. However, there are two types of "hunger," homeostasis hunger and psychological hunger. Homeostasis hunger is a reflexive need to fuel the body for its basic survival; it attempts to maintain the energy balance of the body. In contrast, psychological hunger is merely a craving for food for the sake of it. Eating when you feel this way is sometimes called emotional eating. In the western world, this kind of eating dominates. We eat while doing almost anything from watching TV, watching football, to studying, and so on. We have forgotten what it feels like to experience real hunger, homeostasis hunger. This is where intermittent fasting 16/8 becomes invaluable. It can help you return your body to normal functioning, the way it was originally designed to work. That's great news, isn't it?

The brain is the center from which hunger is controlled. How does the brain know when to trigger hunger pangs? To answer that question, we must look at two major hormones that scientists have found to influence the intake of food. They are leptin and ghrelin. I think it is important here to say that the human body is so complex, with many interacting systems, that it is hard to find a single hormone fully responsible for one function. There are other hormones that play a role in hunger. It is leptin and ghrelin that are the major known role players; hence, our focus on them. Let's talk about the role each plays in hunger.

Leptin

Leptin is produced mainly in the adipose tissue (fat tissue). Small amounts are also secreted by the stomach, mammary epithelium, placenta, and the heart. Leptin is continuously released into the blood circulatory system and crosses the blood-brain barrier. Here, it enters the hypothalamus and binds to the leptin receptors where it signals to the brain the status of the energy stores. If the energy stores are lower than they should be, the hypothalamus triggers more food intake and lower energy expenditure to return the energy stores to normal. Leptin-deficient people tend to become overweight due to increased appetite (and overeating) and decreased physical activity. In the final analysis, leptin serves to maintain the body's energy balance, both in the long-term and short-term.

Ghrelin

Ghrelin is secreted mainly due to an empty stomach. Its main function, research has found, is to stimulate appetite. For example, researchers Klok and colleagues at VU University, Amsterdam, (2007) did a review to determine the role leptin and ghrelin play in the regulation of hunger and body weight in people. They discovered that intravenous injection of ghrelin induces hunger and food intake in humans. Ghrelin levels in the bloodstream vary with time. At about your regular meal time, ghrelin levels peak and after a few hours, drop again. Food intake affects ghrelin levels in the bloodstream as it does leptin levels.

Ghrelin in the bloodstream is transported to the part of the brain called the hypothalamus. Here, it crosses the blood-brain barrier and binds with the ghrelin receptors. The brain "knows" the current amount of ghrelin in the blood and if high, it sends signals to the stomach to activate appetite and hunger pangs. However, if ghrelin levels are low, nothing happens and you won't feel the urge to eat.

As such, ghrelin promotes storage of energy in fat form for the body to use in the event of need, like during an extended period of not eating such as fasting. Ghrelin was also found to stimulate the release of a growth hormone whose function is to reduce body fat and accelerate growth of bones and body mass.

When fasting, the key is more about the frequency and timing of eating. This is not entirely accurate. In their research, Klok et al made a very important observation you should burn on your marvelous mind. Here's what they say, "Not only the size and frequency of meals have an effect on circulating leptin and ghrelin levels, but also the composition of a meal is a determinant of leptin and ghrelin levels in humans." (Klok, Jakobsdottir, & Drent, 2007). So, the kind of food we eat may also impact the effectiveness of our fasting regime. We'll talk more in chapter 6 about food. For now, just keep that at the back of your mind. Let's explore the subject of digestion so we know what happens in our bodies when we eat food.

What is Digestion, Really?

The human body requires energy to carry out its various functions. The major source of this energy for most people is food. However, the body is not equipped to use this food as is. The food must first be converted into suitable forms and the process to do that is called digestion.

Since digestion is a process, it consists of a series of steps or stages. The place where food enters the body is the mouth.

The Mouth

When a person takes in food, it lands first in the mouth. Very little digestion takes place in the mouth; only the mechanical breakdown of food. The tongue mixes the ingested food with saliva for ease of movement to and through to the next step. At the same time, teeth break the larger chunks of food into smaller sizes suitable for the next processing stage. Saliva contains chemicals called enzymes that partially dissolve some of the nutrients contained within the ingested food. The major nutrient dissolved at this stage is starch. Finally, the tongue pushes the chewed food into a relatively long pipe made of muscle called the esophagus.

The Esophagus

No digestion takes place in the esophagus. It simply pushes food forward via the contraction and relaxation of muscles. The process is called peristalsis. In a short time, the food enters the stomach (not tummy!), a sac-like organ found in the rib cage just under the liver.

The Stomach

Immediately as food enters the stomach, digestion begins in earnest. An acid, called gastric acid, dissolves the food while the stomach muscles contract to mix the food. This thorough mixing of food ensures all of the food particles get in contact with digestive juices. At this stage, few nutrients enter the bloodstream. The final product is called chyme, which then enters the small intestine via a small organ called the duodenal bulb.

The Small Intestine

This is the workhorse of the digestion process. A lot of digestion magic happens here. It is here where the large nutrients (macronutrients or macros for short) like carbohydrates, proteins and fats are broken into smaller substances. These smaller substances are small enough to be absorbed into the small intestine via its wall into the bloodstream. Blood delivers these nutrients to various organs of the body where they are used to generate energy in various cells.

The breaking down of the macronutrients into molecules is carried out by enzymes. Bile, from the gall bladder situated on the liver, plays a role in the digestion of fats. It basically emulsifies fats, that is, it turns fat into little droplets that are tiny enough to pass through the barrier between the small intestine and the bloodstream.

Substances called hormones play a vital digestion role as well. They are mainly released by the liver, pancreas, fat cells, and the walls of the intestines.

Finally, any undigested food slowly moves to the last organ of digestion called the colon (also known as the large intestine). The small intestine and colon together can be about nine metres (about 30 feet) in length. They fit in the abdominal cavity (tummy area) in a coiled fashion. Most importantly, they are long by design, so that food stays within the system for a considerable amount of time for optimal absorption of nutrients into the bloodstream.

The Large Intestine

Not much digestion takes place here. The major role of the organ is to prepare waste for elimination from the body. It's also a place where certain bacteria synthesise important vitamins and fiber.

The colon prepares waste by absorbing much of the water from the small intestine. Otherwise, the body would become dehydrated often. And lastly, the waste material is ejected out of the body through the rectum and anus.

As you can see, the brain is really where digestion actually begins. This is important because it can be an opportunity to manipulate how we eat. In fact, we'll go deeper into the workings of the mind (activity of the brain) in chapter 3 because it is such a vital part of weight loss.

The Primary Source of Energy for the Body

Glucose is the primary source of energy for the human body. It is the major product obtained when the body burns carbohydrates like starch. The glucose from carbohydrates is absorbed through the small intestine walls into the bloodstream. A hormone called insulin plays a major role in the absorption of glucose into the cells for energy or storage as glycogen or fat. This essential hormone is secreted by the pancreas. In certain people, cells may become insulin-resistant or the body may produce insufficient insulin. When such situations occur, there may be excessive glucose in the bloodstream, a condition known as hyperglycemia. When the body is unable to control insulin levels, the person may become diabetic.

However, the body is able to produce its own glucose via a process called gluconeogenesis. We'll have a lot to say about this process a little bit later. Excess energy is stored in the body as glycogen in the muscles and liver or as triglycerides in the fat cells. The latter comes in handy during exercise, fasting or keto dieting.

We measure energy in units called kilocalories or kilojoules. Most people are familiar with the term "calories," which works fine for our purpose here. Carbohydrates release about four kilocalories of energy per gram when they are burned. So do the proteins. On the other hand, fats release about 9 kilocalories (over two times more than carbohydrates) per gram. Vitamins, minerals, water, and all other kinds of micronutrients do not provide any sort of energy. They serve other useful purposes. For example, calcium helps in building strong bones.

Finally, and this is important, the human body is remarkably resilient and adaptable. This is exciting because the body can handle a wide variety of diets. And every diet has an effect on human health.

So, when you adopt the intermittent fasting 16/8 lifestyle, remember it's going to affect your health – mainly positively. But the impact could be negative in the first few days of starting it. The good thing is that the negative effects can be neutralised through minor tweaks we'll discuss later, and usually don't last long.

Chapter 2: The Science of Intermittent Fasting

Fasting in general has been around for millennia. People fasted for various reasons including improving memory and thinking, and for religious and political reasons. A good religious example is Ramadan, an Islam fast that lasts for a month. Mahatma Gandhi fasted for political reasons and we know what the outcome of his actions were to the future and lives of Indians.

Just look at what some famous people have said about fasting:

"The best of all medicines is resting and fasting." – Benjamin Franklin

"I fast for greater physical and mental efficiency." – Plato

"Fasting cures diseases, dries up bodily humors, puts demons to flight, gets rid of impure thoughts, makes the mind clearer and the heart purer, the body sanctified, and raises man to the throne of God." – Athenaeus

"Fasting cleanses the soul, raises the mind, subjects one's flesh to the spirit, renders the heart contrite and humble, scatters the clouds of concupiscence, quenches the fire of lust, and kindles the true light of chastity." --Saint Augustine

"Fasting is the first principle of medicine." – Rumi

Looking at the above wisdom, there is no doubt that fasting is essential for effective functioning of the body.

What is Intermittent Fasting 16/8?

First, let's define what fasting is. Well, fasting is a voluntary process where a participant spends a period of time, long or short, without eating food for religious reasons or to promote health. Fasts differ mainly in length of the deprivation of food. Some people fast for 12 hours, others for 24 hours, and still others for over 30 days. These fasting periods are not fixed. One of the common fasting methods is called intermittent fasting 16/8. The practitioner goes through two cycles in a 24-hour period, 16 hours of fasting and 8 hours during which to eat (feeding). The main intention is to induce lower consumption of calories than typical, while focusing entirely on the timing of meals and the frequency of eating.

It is essential to differentiate between fasting and starvation. One key difference is that fasting is voluntary while starvation is involuntary. Starvation occurs when food is denied (usually by lack of food) while the body is in need of sustenance. Fasting, in essence, is principally a house-cleaning technique.

The Science of Intermittent Fasting during the No-Eating Cycle

Most people normally burn carbohydrates to generate energy for effective functioning of their bodies. This practice has caused the body to "forget" to use other, equally efficient, sources of energy. A typical approach to food in the western world almost continuously makes glucose available to the body. There is an unquestionable habit to have breakfast, lunch and dinner in any single day. In addition, we munch on snacks throughout the day. And our busy lifestyles, where working two jobs is not unknown, encourage a high frequency of eating and drinking. As such, our bodies have deviated from the natural way they are meant to work and prefer to almost depend entirely on burning glucose for energy. Unfortunately, this has come at a huge cost as our health has taken a nosedive. Ailments like diabetes and cardiovascular diseases are almost universal, despite advances in medical technology.

For this reason, there is a need to return the body to normal functioning and intermittent fasting 16/8 is a tool to do just that. You see, the cells of the body prefer different kinds of energy sources for full functioning. For example, the brain thrives on energy sourced from burning of glucose or ketones, but can't use fat directly. Yet, heart cells can use fat, ketones and glucose as sources of energy.

During the no-food cycle of intermittent fasting 16/8, carbohydrates as a source of energy get depleted. This happens when blood sugar level drops, often after about 5 hours of taking meals. At this time, insulin levels in the blood also drop. The body's ingenious design counters this drop in an amazing way. What it does is it takes stored glucose in the muscles and the liver called glycogen and converts it to glucose to supply the body's energy needs. However, preference is given to conversion of liver glycogen. Once this glycogen is exhausted, the body takes non-carbohydrate macronutrients like proteins and converts them into glucogenic amino acids (the building blocks of proteins).

Now, these amino acids are eventually converted into glucose for use by the body. This process is called gluconeogenesis, which literally means the generation of new glucose within the body. The proteins used for this purpose primarily come from the muscle, liver cells and to a lesser extent, the renal cortex. This is where the hormone called glucagon becomes very useful as it activates gluconeogenesis. This latter process also occurs when glycerol, a portion of fat, is converted into glucose.

Once gluconeogenesis reaches the end, the blood glucose level drops off once again. The brain, which consumes about 20% of the body's energy, suffers the most from this lack because it does not directly use fatty acids as an energy source. In this state, the body must find a new energy source to continue living. If this doesn't happen, the body will certainly begin to wither and die. Right at this time, fat stored in the body comes to the rescue. Let me make an important point here. Glucose is not an essential nutrient for the human body as we were taught in schools. The reason is that the body can generate glucose by itself, while essential nutrients like magnesium can only be obtained from sources external to the body.

Now, let's see how fat is turned into energy.

How the Body Burns Fat into Energy

When blood glucose levels are low, the body releases low insulin. The low blood glucose message reaches the brain which then tells the body to stop storing fat and glucose. It is at this time that the body begins to burn fat from the fat cells as an energy source, a process termed lipolysis. The by-products of this process are known as ketones and we say the body is in ketosis (this is where the name ketogenic diet comes from).

There are three main kinds of ketones the body releases during lipolysis, namely:

- Beta-hydroxybutyrate: This ketone is found mainly in the blood.
- Acetone: Usually found in breath. For this reason when you are in a ketosis state, it's unlikely to test negative for alcohol using a breathalyzer (breath meter).
- Acetoacetate: It is found mainly in urine.

The ketones mentioned above make it possible to measure whether you are in ketosis or not. This is exciting because it takes the guesswork out of intermittent fasting 16/8. How do we measure ketones? That's a good question. Let's briefly look at how to do that.

There are three ways to measure ketones. We can measure ketones in blood, urine or lungs. When you are in a ketogenic state, your urine contains acetoacetate. To check if you are in keto state, you can use urine strips. They are cheap and very easy to use. However, they are not very accurate because they give qualitative results. This is how you measure the ketones in urine:

- Simply hold a urine strip across your urine stream.
- Remove the strip. The results will appear in 10 to 20 seconds.
- For positive acetoacetate, the strip will become light pink to maroon. The darker the color, the more ketones you have in your

urine. However, the color may be affected if you drink water before testing.

If you want instead, to measure ketones in your breath, you may use a breath meter. It is more accurate than urine strips. The ketone in breath is acetone, which also is found in nail polish remover. It is the reason that nail polish remover has that characteristic smell. Here's how to take the measurements:

- Switch the breath meter on.
- Take a slow and deep breath to fill your lungs with air.
- Put the breath meter in your mouth.
- Exhale fully, emptying the lungs.
- Remove the breath meter from your mouth and wait for a few seconds. The results will appear on the screen of the meter within a few seconds.
- If you want to check for reproducibility of the results, repeat the above process three or four times.

- Finally, record your readings. Go for the highest reading you get because the last bit of air usually contains high amounts of ketones if you are in a ketogenic state.

Measuring ketones this way is essential if you want to stay on intermittent fasting 16/8. If you fast in the night, an ideal time to measure ketones will be in the morning just after you wake up and possibly just before you break the fast. The investment you make on the breath meter will be one of the best ones you can make.

The best way to measure ketones is to use a blood ketone meter. It's more accurate, but more expensive than the urine strips and breath meter. It's the Rolls Royce of ketone measurements. The equipment you need for this are:

- A lancet pen.
- Ketone strips. They can be expensive.
- Blood ketone meter. Usually it can also measure blood glucose.

Simply follow the instructions given in the package on how to use the meter and the strips. When your results are between 0.5 and 3.0 millimoles per litre, you know you are in ketosis.

When you are in a state of ketosis, the fat that the body will burn for energy will come from fat cells. This is good because now you can begin to lose weight as just one of the benefits of ketosis. There are more benefits (we'll discuss this later in depth) for ketosis including:

- It becomes effortless to control your hunger.
- It becomes easier to lose weight and manage it.
- Your mental faculties, like memory, improve.
- You sleep better, probably like a healthy baby.
- You gain better control of blood sugar and restore insulin sensitivity.
- You lower inflammation levels meaning less internal infections.

It is obvious that once you realize the benefits of ketosis, your medical bills will go down, don't you think so? Isn't that exciting news? Sure it is.

There's confusion in the marketplace whether ketosis is safe or not. The bulk of the fears stem from the fact that high ketone levels in certain special cases can cause a life-threatening ketogenic state called ketoacidosis. It is essential, then, to talk about this condition to clear the air.

What is Ketoacidosis?

As the body keeps producing ketones, their concentration increases in the blood. There are certain cases that this can happen when the blood sugar level is too high for far too long. When these two conditions occur at the same time, a condition called ketoacidosis occurs. It can be life-threatening if allowed to linger.

Now, how does the body reach a state of ketoacidosis? That's a great question.

You see, the body can reach a point where it is unable to control blood sugar levels. This is an indication that the body is releasing insufficient insulin into the bloodstream. Insulin opens the cell gates to allow glucose to enter and burn as energy. This condition is common in people who have type 1 diabetes and whose bodies make barely enough insulin for normal functioning.

When the body is not getting glucose, it assumes there's a shortage of this important energy source. So, it instructs the cells to use alternative fuels. Eventually, the body begins to burn fat, thereby producing ketones. The amount of ketones keeps increasing because the body requires energy all the time. If the ketone amount reaches about 20 millimoles, a life-threatening situation occurs. The person may even fall into a coma. It's important to emphasize that this occurs mostly among type 1 diabetic patients. It is perhaps these people who should continuously measure their glucose levels and also measure ketone levels in their blood a few times a day to avoid uncontrolled ketosis.

In type 2 diabetics, who are insulin-dependent, this condition is rare. The reason is that these patients can control their blood glucose levels and thus prevent a condition of high blood glucose and high ketone levels. As for non-diabetic people, the condition is unheard of. So, be rest assured that it is safe to go on intermittent fasting 16/8 even if you have type 2 diabetes. If you have doubts, consult a physician who understands how ketosis works. Usually, a family physician is untrained on nutrition matters and may advise you erroneously about intermittent fasting 16/8 (or fasting in general). So, choose your physician carefully.

There's a clear difference between nutritional ketosis and ketoacidosis. Nutritional ketosis occurs only when there are low blood sugar levels present. In contrast, ketoacidosis occurs when both blood sugar and ketone bodies are high. It is for this reason that during ketosis, you must ensure that your blood sugar levels are under control. That's why it's important to measure your glucose levels regularly when you are in ketosis or even use continuous glucose meters.

Chapter 3: The Real Core Reason a Majority of People Fail to Lose Weight

People go on diets for various reasons. When the International Food Information Council (IFIC) Foundation surveyed 1009 Americans in March 2018, they discovered interesting facts. For example, they found that cardiovascular health came out tops when researchers asked these people what it was they were interested in getting from food. Surprisingly, it was not to be satiated or full, as we may have expected. See the figure below:

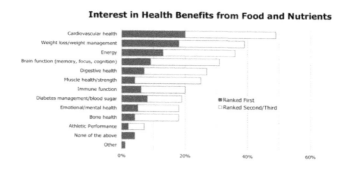

Figure 3: Results of a survey to find out why people go on diet

Second on the list was weight loss and weight management. This is not surprising because obesity is one of the main health challenges today's society is facing. Third was for energy purposes. We know it's essential to have floods of energy to live meaningful lives. And fourth, these people picked brain function, which means memory improvement, focus and thinking. The latter, as far as we know, is the highest function human beings are capable of. It's appropriate to have this aspect of our lives as one of the reasons to choose certain foods. And lastly, on position five, the reason to diet was given as for digestive health.

Arguably, weight loss and weight management cause a large number of people sleepless nights. It's not surprising that the same study revealed that people adopted new eating patterns to lose weight. See the figure below for a full listing of the reasons for adopting new eating patterns.

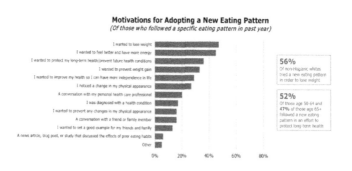

Motivations for Adopting a New Eating Pattern
(Of those who followed a specific eating pattern in past year)

I wanted to lose weight
I wanted to feel better and have more energy
I wanted to protect my long-term health/prevent future health conditions
I wanted to prevent weight gain
I wanted to improve my health so I can have more independence in life
I noticed a change in my physical appearance
A conversation with my personal health care professional
I was diagnosed with a health condition
I wanted to prevent any changes in my physical appearance
A conversation with a friend or family member
I wanted to set a good example for my friends and family
A news article, blog post, or study that discussed the effects of poor eating habits
Other

0%   20%   40%   60%   80%

56%
Of non-Hispanic whites tried a new eating pattern in order to lose weight

52%
Of those age 50-64 and 47% of those age 65+ followed a new eating pattern in an effort to protect long-term health

Figure 4: Major reasons people adopt new diets

The reason is simple. You see, overweight or obese people have a higher chance of getting chronic ailments like type 2 diabetes, heart diseases, and hypertension (high blood pressure). These diseases can completely change a person's life. For example, you become forced to avoid certain dishes you like. If you have type 2 diabetes, your sexual activities may be immensely affected. This is like getting one of your body parts severed and life may become less fulfilling.

Despite people eating certain foods to manage their weight, data abounds that suggest a big chunk who go on diet fail. For example, an article in the UK's *Mail Online* shares the results of a survey of over 2,000 Britons done by Alpro, a company that promotes plant-based eating. This survey revealed that two out of every five people on a diet quit in the first seven days! And that only one keeps going strong beyond one month.

But why?

There are many reasons given for this. A close scrutiny boils the reasons down to people's behaviors – they don't support being on a strict diet. Most people make a serious mistake of trying to fight their behaviors through their willpower. This powerful mental faculty works for only a few because the majority of us have never received any training to develop this mental prowess. Hence, many tap out of chosen diets too early before they have enough time to work their magic. Don't worry, I'm not going to train you to develop yours. There is a mental trick you can play to subtly and effectively change your eating behavior to match your weight desire. There is a simple solution. But before I give you the solution, there's something else you need to know and understand about how the mind works.

Shortcut Knowledge on How Human Nature Affects Diet Plans

You see, human beings are creatures of habit, and habit is the body's mechanism to make routine work almost automatic. For example, blinking an eye is a habit as it happens almost without notice. Habits are a key to tweaking certain behaviors that may have led us to side-step healthy living. They can make or break your marvelous diet ideas. So, how do we modify them to support our diet goals and dreams?

It starts with understanding how habits are formed. This is where the human mind comes in. You may be aware that your mind works in pictures. For example, if I say the word, "chocolate," what do you see on the screen of your mind? Some chocolate picture, isn't it? Probably a certain kind of chocolate you like best or hate most! If, instead, I say the word, "dog," what comes on the screen of your mind? A dog, of course. I'm sure you get the idea now.

Here's something important; the words I mentioned above, chocolate and dog, mean nothing to someone who has *never* seen the objects they represent. It follows that for your mind to recognize something, its picture must first be stored in it. And for it to be stored, somebody or something deliberately or unconsciously must put it in the mind. For most of us, ideas were implanted in our minds whilst we were still below the age of seven. At that period of our lives, the formative period, our brains were flooded with neutrons so we could learn a lot more information in a shorter time to improve our survival chances.

Unfortunately, some of the ideas we picked up weren't necessarily helpful to us. Take for example the story of breakfast. Who said it must be eaten in the morning? The word "breakfast," is composed of two separate words, "break" and "fast." Thus, breakfast literally means to break a fast. And breaking a fast can happen anytime during the day, not necessarily in the morning. We rarely question a lot of what we do and this is partly why deadly conditions like obesity are skyrocketing throughout the world. Anyway, let's continue to see how we can reverse this unfortunate situation for weight loss purposes,

The pictures we have in our minds drive our behaviors. This means you must store the picture you want to see of yourself when your diet is successful in your mind before your weight loss program becomes sustainable. It is here we must learn how your mind works.

Over the years, people have discovered a simple way the mind works to bring results in our lives. Two people come to mind, Joseph Murphy, author of *The Power of Your Subconscious Mind* and a chiropractor by the name of Dr. Thurman Fleet. But they themselves got their ideas from studying other cultures, especially from the Orient. At any rate, the mind works at two primary levels in conjunction with the body. Here's how it works:

The Conscious Level

This is the part that interacts with the surroundings (environment). The senses (eyes, ears, skin, nose, and tongue) are the agents that connect the conscious mind with the environment. When a message comes to this part from the environment, it is either accepted or rejected. It's more like a sieve. The rejected information is thrown away. Such information won't affect a person's behavior. On the flipside, the accepted information moves further to the next part of the mind called the subconscious level.

The Subconscious Level

The suffix 'sub' means below. So subconscious means below the conscious. This means we are not able to notice the exact operations of this part or level of the mind. For example, we don't fully know how the mind stores vast information in our brain. It just happens.

This part receives messages from the conscious level. It has no ability to reject and thus can only accept. This means what comes here is considered as gospel, whether it is right or wrong. When we are born, our conscious is undeveloped and so most of what comes to us simply enters the subconscious almost freely. You can compare the subconscious with a writable compact disc. It does not block you from saving information on it and doesn't choose for you what information to burn on it. I'm sure you get the idea. Our memories and emotions are housed in this deductive part of our minds. When the Bible says, "As a man thinketh in his heart," it is referring to this section of the mind. Once information successfully enters this part, it is sent to the relevant body parts for execution. Most people fail to lose weight permanently because they've never changed the image of themselves in this part of the mind. So, any attempt to lose weight causes the subconscious to work to regain the weight to match the picture in the mind.

The Body

The body is the instrument of the subconscious level of the mind. It simply does what the subconscious tells it to do without question. Once you do some act, there's a reaction from the environment and the reaction is what we call results. This means if the subconscious is not programmed to support your diet plans, chances are that you'll find it hard to follow your meal plans. And thus the body will NOT do what you said you want (lose weight for example). And that can be discouraging indeed. But don't worry. I'll show you how to get your subconscious to work with you, not against you, like it does with most other people.

As you can see, working to directly change your behavior is like pushing water uphill because you depend primarily on the conscious part of the mind. It requires tons of willpower to get this part to do things the way you want. You are actually fighting your nature, and you can easily give up and many do when trying to lose weight. If you had a choice, would you choose to push a big rock up or down a slope? For sure, you'll choose down the slope all the time. Why then try to work against your biology? Willpower is good but it's tiring, especially to the mind. The brain, a tool the mind mostly uses, prefers to conserve energy. It's stingy.

How do we side-step this natural set-up of the human organism? It's easy. The process should take you less than ten minutes daily for a few weeks. All it requires is something called persistence and the ability to follow routine. But persistence is a by-product of something we call a goal because without a goal, there's no reason to persist. Without persistence, your body is likely to stay overweight or obese or you'll be a friend to chronic diseases like diabetes. You may also remain in fatigue mode, with little energy. Here's an important question.

Why Do You Want to Lose Weight?

This is a great question, isn't it? Many people who decide to go on intermittent fasting 16/8 miss this. And they quickly sign off from the diet regime they themselves initially decided to follow. This is tragic, don't you think so?

To succeed on a diet plan, it's essential to make a committed decision, not a mere wish. A committed decision happens when you emotionally and intellectually know why you are doing something. If you know why you are dieting or you want to diet and you are emotionally connected to the idea, that's great. But if you are unsure what your reason for dieting is, read on.

Imagine for a moment that your body is the way you want it to be. How does it look? How do you feel when walking in a shopping mall or at work? How do you feel when friends and family compliment you on your well-shaped body? What kinds of clothes are you wearing most of the time? How do you feel when people ask you how you did it? How does it feel when your mind is thinking clearly and your memory is in high gear? How does it feel when you stay energetic throughout the day when others next to you feel sluggish?

Now, write the answers to all the above questions on a piece of clean paper. These questions made you "see" who you wish to become. I'm sure it feels great, doesn't it? Of course it does, and that's good. Now, this image of your new you must be committed to the subconscious level of your mind or else you will likely regain any weight you lose. You want your body and mind to align so that they take you to your desired body almost automatically -- without the tiring conscious effort. Perhaps you also want to improve your health. That also can happen once you have stored your new image in your subconscious.

How Do You Store This New Picture in Your Subconscious?

It's simple. Take that little piece of paper and make two copies of it. Stick one copy at home in a room where you can see it often and place another copy right where you can see it often at your workplace. Keep the third copy with you all the time and read it immediately when you wake up in the morning as well as in the afternoon after eating your lunch. And lastly, read it again in the evening just before you retire to bed. The reason for this is that in the mornings and evenings, your conscious lets the guard down and you can then easily pass this new image to the subconscious. In addition, when you frequently present an image to the conscious, it finally assumes the information must be important. And it finally lets it percolate into the subconscious so it can be acted on automatically.

This is the most practical way psychologists and ancient masters of the mind have discovered human beings can reprogram themselves the way they want. Perhaps a better approach could be to record the information on the piece of paper using your phone or some recording device and then listening to it several times a day. Repetition is the mother of learning. I'm sure you know this already.

The subconscious part will tell the body to do the necessary things to make the image a reality without you realizing it. If you take this little lesson on how to impress the image you want into your subconscious, you'll understand, intellectually and emotionally, what Dr. Maxwell Maltz, (1960), who was a plastic surgeon and authored *Psycho-cybernetic Principles: a new way to get more living out of life*, meant when he said these words: "The most important psychological discovery of this century is the discovery of the self-image." Whether we realize it or not, each of us carries about with us a mental blueprint or picture of ourselves." And that picture guides what we do with our lives.

How long this process takes depends on the individual. Each of our mental make-up is different. To some it may take a few days and with others it may take perhaps a few weeks. And still to others it may take months (perhaps 3 months or so). But if it gives you the kind of body you want, does it really matter how long it takes? Haven't you known people who kept going after what they wanted even when faced with huge obstacles? I'm sure you do. So, you have no excuse for NOT doing this exercise.

Lastly, I applaud you for reading this material until the end. It shows you are eager to achieve the diet results you want. Most people are quick to jump to the "how" part and meal plans without first setting a strong foundation for consistent use of the given strategies; they then wonder why they lose weight quickly and regain it back within a short time, like some of The Biggest Loser contestants.

Now we are ready to look at research that rocked the world of medicine and nutrition. This information has opened people's eyes about diets and nutrition and it will help you look at diets in a new perspective. We lived with this myth for too long and it is time the world knew we were fed lies.

Chapter 4: Myth – There's a Common Diet for Everyone

Why is it that two people can both start the same diet program at the same time and yet one wins and another fails? The same goes for the intermittent fasting 16/8 protocol. Some people lose weight and keep it off permanently, while others don't seem to be winning at all. For example, here is a story of an intermittent faster who was concerned that she regained weight after trying the protocol. Let's listen to her: "I'm 3 weeks into intermittent fasting. I'm a female of 32 and 5 foot 4 inches tall. I started intermittent fasting at 194 pounds and followed the 16/8 method. I also exercised several times a week. Initially, my weight dropped to 189lbs, but I'm now back to weighing 192lbs. I'm seriously losing hope. Please help."

Yet there are people who have found phenomenal success with the same kind of weight loss regime. Like this one: "I'm 2 months into intermittent fasting 16/8 and I've gone from 417 pounds to 385 pounds. I've just recently added cardio to my routine and I must say that I feel better than I've felt in years. Intermittent fasting has been a literal life saver for me."

There you have it. Two people, same weight loss regime, yet one feels down while another is over the moon. How can this be? This chapter goes to science to find the answers. Yes, some doctors, weight loss writers and intermittent fasting researchers may know what they believe are causes for weight loss failure, but there's more to it that is not obvious. And we'll tear open the veil and expose the science behind nutrition, which is essential in any weight loss intervention.

One of the biggest weaknesses of human beings, including learned brethren like scientists, have a tendency to generalize. You see, generalizations create groups which can be described in a few words. For example, women generally refer to men as dogs on matters of promiscuity. But, are all men really dogs as these women suggest? Certainly not. Another example. Biologists often classify species according to similar characteristics called taxonomies. But within a given taxonomy there are countless differences amongst the members.

Generalization is really an outgrowth of people's tendency to take shortcuts to save the energy required to think hard and to ferret out all the details. It is a hard task to find as much details as possible on a given subject, one very few people ever dream of doing.

No wonder there's a large stock of books, videos and articles pregnant with pre-defined diet plans. These sources *assume* people are the same. This probably impacts whether people who go on diets become successful or fail and perhaps we shouldn't be shocked when only two out every five people who go on a diet fail within seven days.

There are several factors that influence the effectiveness of a diet, including what you eat during the feeding cycle of intermittent fasting, besides the actual food and calories consumed. Yet, there are experts out there who focus almost exclusively on the actual diet and ignore other factors. They erroneously forget that human life and the human body are complex.

To emphasize the dangers of generalizations, let's dive into a diet-related study conducted in Israel by Zeevi and his colleagues. The researchers were interested in designing a system that could be used to personalize nutrition by predicting blood glucose responses to food intake. This study, published on page 1079 of a prestigious journal called *Cell*, revealed interesting facts regarding factors that affect blood glucose levels. It is widely known that blood glucose level is a risk factor that can be linked to major diseases such as:

- Obesity.
- Cardiovascular diseases.
- Hypertension.
- Hypertriglyceridemia (excessive fatty acids).
- Non-alcoholic fatty liver diseases.
- Diabetes.
- Chronic metabolic diseases.

Therefore, controlling and maintaining normal blood glucose levels is essential because it is the key to prevent diseases associated with hyperglycemia (excessive blood glucose levels). Perhaps we ignore implementing prevention methods because our society is used to dealing with symptoms of diseases rather than actual causes. Just check how huge is the pharmaceutical industry and you'll get what I mean. And this industry hires some of the most astute copywriters, psychologists, psychiatrists, and other specialists to create marketing messages that easily influence us to buy their drugs, some helpful and some hazardous to our health.

What this study by Zeevi *et al* (2015) did was recruit 800 healthy and pre-diabetic people whose age ranged from 18 to 70. The researchers also wanted to establish if people would respond the same way or differently if they ate the same food.

These experts then gave the participants carefully carbohydrate-controlled meals, totaling 5,107 and measured, for each participant, the following for a week:

- Blood parameters like blood sugar levels.
- Physical activities.
- Anthropometrics such as body mass index.
- Gut microbiota (micro-organisms in the digestive tract, especially the large intestine).
- Stool samples (taken to measure these microorganisms).
- Self-reported lifestyle behaviors.

Blood glucose was continuously measured using subcutaneous sensors every five minutes for 46,898 meals. This means over 1.5 million blood glucose readings were taken over the week of the trial. Most importantly, the participants were asked to follow their normal daily routines and dietary habits. This was an important idea because the results were intended to closely resemble normal daily life situations, not laboratory-controlled life. The only exception was the first meal of the day, which the researchers provided. This controlled meal consisted of 50 grams of available carbohydrates. By the way, a day's worth of ketogenic-type meals consists of about 50 grams of carbohydrates or less. (A side note: Researchers always take baseline measurements at the start of a significant study such as this one to identify changes that may take place during the investigation).

What did the researchers discover, you may wonder? The answer stunned even these learned scientists. They discovered that the level of glucose in the blood varied for different people even if they ate the same kind of food. Interestingly, each person's response to the same meal was the same on different days as shown in the figure below. This means when you eat a certain food regularly, it will impact you the same way day after day. See the figure below for the actual measurements plotted on a graph to show you the pattern.

C

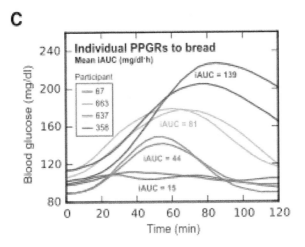

Figure 5: Post-meals blood responses of study participants

Compare, for example, participant numbers 15 and 139. Just look at how the blood glucose levels for participant 139 as opposed to that of participant 15. The two measurements of blood glucose for the same participant were about the same on different days though she ate the same meal. However, there is a vast difference of about 100 mg/dL post meal glucose levels between the two participants. This study suggests that every person who goes on a diet should measure (probably continuously where possible) their blood glucose content.

These experts predicted the factors they believed could be at the center of this variability and they include genetic factors, lifestyle, insulin sensitivity, exocrine pancreatic and glucose transporters activity levels. One other factor is gut microbiota, which has been associated with obesity, glucose intolerance, type 2 diabetes, hyperlipidemia and insulin resistance.

The discovery that blood glucose varies for different people after eating the same kind of meal offers interesting implications. For example, it means any person can actually discover a suitable meal to help them control blood glucose and effortlessly get the kind of body they want. What does this mean to you with respect to intermittent fasting 16/8? In short, it means you are not just going to eat any food you want, as many articles and some intermittent fasting books suggest. You are going to establish the kind of food that will help you burn your body fat until you hit your target weight level. The way to do that is to measure your post meal blood glucose, say one hour, after eating. Once you do this for a number of varieties of meals, you should know the kind of recipes ideal for YOU to lose weight.

Not every meal you eat during your feeding cycle will help you to lose weight. Some of the food may actually promote weight gain. We'll explain in chapter 6 the kind of food favorable for successful weight loss using intermittent fasting 16/8. For now, just burn it in your mind that you are a unique individual, responding differently to the same food as the person next to you.

There were more interesting findings from the study we introduced above. The figure below illustrates how two participants responded to glucose and bread. Interestingly, you would expect both participants to have high levels of blood glucose after consuming glucose. Strangely, that was not the case. Participant 468 responded as expected (wouldn't you expect eating sugar to increase your blood glucose?) but participant 663 responded in the opposite way. The blood glucose level actually was lower. Interesting, isn't it?

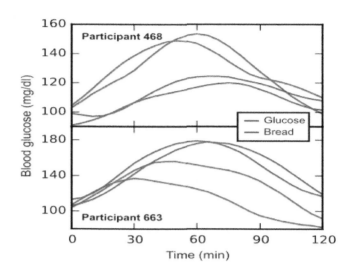

Figure 6: Blood glucose response of two
participants after taking bread and glucose

It just goes to further show that people's bodies are complex. Assuming people will respond the same way to the same diet is clearly a mistake. This same study also discovered that factors like gut micro-organisms and lifestyle influence blood glucose levels. So, in considering weight loss via intermittent fasting 16/8, it's not enough to merely fast and modify your nutrition, but to also change your lifestyle. A sedentary lifestyle may likely not help you lose much weight.

Perhaps you'll say we cannot make up our minds from just one research study, whether there is a one-size-fits-all diet or not. I totally understand. Hence, we'll look at more science-based evidence to ensure this idea sits snugly in your long-term memory. But first, let me tell you a story of a girl who battled with losing weight in the intermittent fasting 16/8 style.

This cute girl has been in intermittent fasting now for over 2 years. Her main reason for starting intermittent fasting 16/8 was to shed some body fat and liked this protocol because she felt it was easy for her. She could easily fit the protocol into her normal daily life without restricting her lifestyle. She especially liked the fact that you can set your fasting and feeding cycles anyway you like. Unfortunately, in the beginning this young woman battled to get any headway with her weight loss program. It turns out she was making a few mistakes, the first one of which many people make. As we showed above, not every meal is suitable for everyone. We even have different metabolic rates; we burn calories at different rates. At any rate, this girl chose 12:00 noon to 20:00 as her feeding time. However, instead of eating enough food to satisfy her hunger, she consumed extra food to meet her emotional eating habits. She even ate protein bars as if they were about to go out of production. No wonder she began gaining weight, instead of losing it, and reversed her previously hard-won weight loss gains. Fortunately, she made a few tweaks and shed off the weight she mistakenly gained. We'll detail the kind of food to eat in chapter 6 for a successful intermittent fasting 16/8 protocol.

Now, if you think the one study we talked about above does not convince you that people respond differently to an identical meal, let me offer you another study. This research, and its phase two is being done as I write this, confirms what we said above. The study involved 1100 people from the U.S. and the U.K. Amongst these participants, there were 240 pairs of twins. The researchers wanted to know, as in the above study, if people respond the same way to the same diet and they planned to check the effect of genetic, metabolic, metagenomics, and meals on after-meals glucose levels, insulin and triacylglycerol. Out of the results, they wished to build a computer algorithm to predict an individual's response to food and thus help with food selection. The results of this research were released during the American Society for Nutrition conference in June 2019.

Participants were given pre-formulated meals for two weeks, while during this process, the researchers measured blood glucose levels, insulin levels, and fat levels. They also analyzed the micro-organisms in the gut. Additionally, the sleep and exercise patterns of the participants were tracked.

The findings matched those of the Israeli study. They discovered that one person could have high blood glucose levels after eating a given meal while a person close by measured lower blood glucose levels even if they have eaten identical meals.

These studies provide enough evidence to suggest people respond differently to the same meals. However, the researchers in both studies do not know for sure why people respond differently to the same meal, except the hypothesis we mentioned in the first study above. For you and me, the most important takeaway from this work is that each one of us has a unique diet that works for them. So, the general nutrition guidelines governments dish out may work for some people, but not all of the nation's citizens. This puts the responsibility for your health right on your capable shoulders if you want to become and stay healthy.

So, it's essential for you to find the diet that works for you. And the best method, if a method at all, is trial and error. Try combinations of meals while measuring your glucose levels and soon you'll discover dishes that are good for your unique body.

We are now ready to dig into the subject of how to get started safely with intermittent fasting 16/8. And if you're ready, let's dive in.

Chapter 5: How to Get Started with Intermittent Fasting 16/8

The purpose of intermittent fasting 16/8 is to enter the body into fat-burning mode and lose weight and get other benefits too, like a lower risk of developing high blood pressure. However, not everyone can benefit from fasting and so, it's important to know if fasting is safe for you. Before we discuss how to get started with intermittent fasting, let's talk about who shouldn't fast.

Don't Fast if...

You are Under the Age of 18

I know a girl who was 17 in 2017, who participated in the Muslim fast of Ramadan. She was in the 12th grade and she attended classes regularly during the month. All she had throughout the day was water. I remember seeing her carrying a water bottle wherever she went while at school. You are probably wondering why then do I say under 18's shouldn't fast? This girl was born in a Muslim family and began fasting from an early age for durations her body could manage as per Muslim requirements.

But for ordinary children, fasting is not the norm and shouldn't be. At this age, the child is still in his or her growth spurt and fasting makes nutrients necessary for growth unavailable. And this may later affect the child's cognitive and motor development. However, it will not be catastrophic if a child misses a meal or two. The most important thing for the child is to eat healthy food, not junk food, which packs the body with foreign, toxic matter.

You Have an Eating Disorder

Eating disorders like anorexia originate as a result of the fear of gaining weight. Such people tend to tightly control the amount of food they eat and may also exercise rigorously to keep weight off. Irrespective of how much weight they lose, anorexians maintain the fear of gaining weight. In most cases, these people are usually underweight and therefore should not fast for their safety.

You Have Less than 4% Body Fat

When body fat is less than 4%, you may be in starvation or malnutrition mode. In this state, it is not advisable to fast. Here's why. During the fast, your body may begin to burn proteins in the muscle tissues to keep the body alive. This will certainly weaken the body and ultimately you may be unable to even move. This phenomenon is called wasting, and is an unhealthy condition to be in.

You are Breastfeeding

To provide the child with the necessary nutrients, your body requires healthy food. In a fasted mode you won't be able to produce the right kind of milk during the fasting cycle and your child may not get the right nutrients. This would certainly affect the growth of your child. I'm sure this is not what you want and therefore choose not to fast. If you absolutely must fast, perhaps putting your toddler on baby formula may be the best alternative.

You are Pregnant

The fetus requires nourishment from nutrients to support optimal growth. Fasting cuts off supply of these nutrients to you and ultimately, to the fetus. Inadequate supply of the nutrients may lead to harm or even death during this important phase of fetus development. To give birth to a healthy new-born, avoid fasting. I'm sure since pregnancy only lasts for 9 months, you can stick it out. But remember fasting is not a good thing to do when breastfeeding.

If You have Any of these Conditions, Do this First

There are certain conditions that make fasting risky while facing them. For this reason, it is absolutely vital to seek medical advice from a qualified physician before entering into a fast.

These conditions include:

Gout

This is a condition that occurs when you have high levels of uric acid in the joints. People with this illness tend to rely on medication to maintain low levels of uric acid. The body eliminates uric acid out of the body via the passing of urine. Now, during fasting, the amount of urine drops and thus uric acid may build up in the body. It is not known how much uric acid the body can tolerate before the situation becomes dire. However, one body of research that studied the effect of Ramadan on patients with gout found no significant increase in uric acid during fasting. In fact, the researchers found that serum uric acid only increased from 7.92 mg/dL to 8.11 mg/dL during the whole month of fasting.

But you must be careful because people may respond differently to the same diet situation. So, it's better to seek medical advice before beginning with intermittent fasting 16/8 if you have gout.

Taking Medications

Certain medications work well only in a full stomach and this is not possible if you are fasting. Medications that can cause problems when fasting include aspirin (used for thinning of blood), metformin (to control blood glucose for type 2 diabetes patients) and supplements of iron and magnesium.

You Have Diabetes

Medications prescribed for diabetic patients are usually administered per the diet the individual follows. So, when going into a fast, there may be a need to change the medications to suit your new diet program. As such, always see your physician before entering into any fasting program, including intermittent fasting 16/8.

Getting Started with Intermittent Fasting 16/8

Now that you know whether you can fast or not, it's time to go into the actual process of intermittent fasting 16/8. All we have done so far is merely foreplay; the real action begins now. But what we did was necessary to prepare you for exactly this stage.

To succeed with intermittent fasting 16/8, especially as a beginner, it is vital to start small, to take baby steps. This is in accordance with the way change occurs. Even Newton, the English mathematician and physicist, observed this phenomenon and coined a law called *Newton's First Law of Motion*. It says, "A body at rest or moving with uniform velocity will continue with its state of motion unless acted on by a net force." What Newton says here is that it takes massive energy to change the state of motion of an object. So it is with changing human behavior. To make a change of behavior, it takes a significant amount of strength. But there is a simpler way out.

Begin small. There are a number of benefits you get by approaching intermittent fasting 16/8 in this way.

- Small steps require very little effort. All you do is to align your fast with your daily routine so it becomes almost effortless to start.
- Fasting will appear easy to your mind. You see, the mind tends to exaggerate the fasting process. It makes it look like an undoable chore. I'm going to suggest you begin by making a small change daily, unlike to expect you to fast, right from the start with a 16-hour fast. Once you get started, it will become effortless to continue.
- It is easier to make small commitments than large ones. This suffocates the negative chatter that floods our minds and so, it won't make a big deal of the small change you make. This will enable you to slowly

expand your comfort zone. Remember that willpower is simply a fight against the size of the task at hand. The bigger the task, the more willpower you require to get started. However, a small task needs just enough willpower to get you started. Once you get started, you'll be astonished to experience higher energy levels and begin to take bigger steps.

Now, let's get started with your intermittent fasting 16/8 protocol.

1. Choose your fasting and feeding periods. As an example, we'll take it your schedule requires you to skip breakfast. And we'll take it your dinner takes place at 20:00. You are going to begin your fast today after dinner. This then becomes your day 1 of fasting. After dinner, avoid opportunities to snack such as while watching TV with your loved ones. This is probably going to be your biggest challenge in the beginning. However, have a bottle of water nearby to

drink in the event you feel like eating a snack or two. Your fast will last until the following day at 8:00 a.m.

2. It's now the end of your day 1 of fasting and you can have breakfast at 8:00a.m. By this time, you have successfully completed a 12-hour fast. And it was effortless because most of it you did while fast asleep. At this point, you have not hit the 16 hour fasting and 8 hour feeding cycle yet. You are at this moment sitting at a 12-hour feeding period and a 12-hour fasting period. You should celebrate this achievement if you hadn't done it before, you know. You can have other meals and dinner during the next 12 hours. After dinner at 20:00, begin with your second fasting day.

3. On day 2, repeat what you did on day 1, but delay your breakfast by one hour. In other words, have your breakfast at 9:00 a.m. and dinner at the same time, 20:00. You have now completed a 13-hour fast and a second day of fasting.

4. On day 3, repeat what you did on day 2, but have breakfast at 10:00 a.m. and dinner at 20:00. Time to celebrate because you have just hit 14 hours of fasting. Is it difficult? Sure, it's not. If it feels a bit challenging, remind yourself why you decided to fast in the first place. That will help you keep going. Be your best cheerleader.

5. On day 4, repeat day 3 and eat breakfast and dinner at 11:00 a.m. and 20:00 respectively. Now, your fasting duration is....eh....eh.... let's see, it's 15 hours. Great work. You have now successfully negotiated your day of intermittent fasting. You have just one hour left to hit the 16 to 8 fasting and eating split. Let's give it another shot.

6. On day 5, repeat day 4 plus have breakfast (maybe we should call it lunch, don't you think so?) at 12:00 noon and have dinner at your usual 20:00 time. By this time, you have already beaten the breakfast meal. And voila, you now have fasted for 16 hours perhaps for the first time. Congratulations!

7. Day 6 is merely a repeat of day 5 until fasting this way becomes your new way of life. Now, watch yourself as the weight disappears, and your energy levels get a significant boost. By this time, you may be sleeping much better than before you began fasting. You now have experienced firsthand what the Chinese meant when they said, "The journey of a thousand miles begins with the first step" or the Japanese kaizen. Remember to keep reading the little paper on which you wrote your primary reasons for intermittent fasting.

As you progressed with your fast, you may have observed certain unusual things about your body. Don't worry, the fast is (was) doing its job. Let me share with you what you may experience as you fast, so your mind is at ease.

What Happens as Fasting Progresses

For most people, intermittent fasting 16/8 may appear unpleasant. Now, tell me, which is more unpleasant, staying overweight (or even sick) or house-cleaning your body for a healthy lifestyle? You know, we tend to have the wrong image about fasting and this may make fasting distressful. But the suffering we anticipate is really not about fasting. It is due mainly to thinking about the absence of the niceties of life like coffee, a few beers, fries, pizzas, chocolate bars, and so on. The thought of missing these treats haunts us.

In the early days of fasting, it is not unknown to feel a consistent demand for food. This is normal. Other unpleasant experiences may include headaches, dizziness, nausea, vomiting and other symptoms. This happens because the body is responding to a sudden withdrawal of habitual stimulants, and it's a sign of a body that's in bad shape.

Fasting is like stopping smoking. A non-smoker does not suffer from a smoking fast, but a smoker who fasts from cigarette suffers greatly. Why? The smoker is actually not suffering because of the fast itself, but as a result of prior smoking. Smoking had become a habit, despite being bad to the health of the smoker. If due to the distress, our friend stops with smoking fasts, the distress of abstaining disappears immediately. But one thing is for sure, he or she will continue to suffer the negative effects of smoking, and make it even more difficult to stop in the future. Fasting, in the beginning, is like stopping smoking. The distress of abstaining from eating can bring with it nervousness, gastric stress, insomnia, and so on. This tends to be common in people whose bodies are unhealthy. Hence, the need for a fast. There are some signs that indicate that the fast is working its magic for such an individual. For example:

- The tongue may become coated.
- Teeth may become pasty.
- Breath tends to become foul due to formation of ketones.
- Taste may become bad.

Brushing of teeth may help neutralize the smell and clean the teeth to remove foreign material. The indicators mentioned above are evidence that fasting is working and therefore, we should welcome those signs. Take this quote by Austin in 1922 as it is relevant here: "A very good test indeed of a so-called perfectly healthy person's state of health is the effect produced in him or her by missing one or more meals. If the tongue begins to get coated and the breath foul and the individual feels seedy and out of sorts, it is proof positive that the state of health is not as good as it was supposed to be."

Now that you are forewarned about what may happen in the beginning of intermittent fasting and you know how to get started, it's time to talk about the food that is good during fasting.

Chapter 6: What to Eat during Intermittent Fasting 16/8

Remember the girl we talked about earlier in the book who lost and then regained her weight? As you may recall, she thought she could munch on anything she wanted during her cycle, only to discover she was completely wrong. That's kind of a sad story, one I believe shouldn't happen to anyone, including you. So, what should you feed on and still keep your weight where you want? Hang on to me as I'm about to take you through the different kinds of food that can help you become full while maintaining your health and losing weight. I'm not going to tell you which specific meals to eat because I don't know exactly what your preferences are and to what level your body tolerates those meals. All I'll do is present nutritional and health information for a select number of food items from which you may make your choices. It is important to remember though, that your meals should contain proteins, carbohydrates and fats in the proportion your body can tolerate.

1. Berries

These include raspberries, blueberries and strawberries. They are available in a number of different colors such as red, black and yellow with each color pregnant with a unique combination of vitamins, minerals, flavonoids and antioxidants. The latter is very useful because they help the body fight free radicals which are associated with inflammation and other health issues. They further contribute to the health of the brain and the overall nervous system. It is advisable to feed on fresh or frozen berries because they don't contain added sugar.

Berries also contain fiber, the holy grail of a clean large intestine. Besides this, fiber is known to help reduce cholesterol levels, management of blood pressure and support weight loss. There are also nutrients such as potassium that help with blood clotting due to some injury. Potassium also helps with balancing of electrolytes in the body, may lower the chances of heart disease and stroke, and assists with reducing the risk of forming kidney stones and bone loss as you age.

In 2010, a team of scientists wanted to investigate the effect of low pH and high antioxidant levels in the killing of three cell types. What they did was treat the stomach, colon, and breast cancer cells with a berry extract solution and also with a solution mixture of hydrochloric acid and ascorbic acid of same pH. Results were astonishing to say the least. The ascorbic acid solution killed only 10% of the stomach, colon, and breast cancer cells. On the other hand, the berry extract terminated over 90% of the cancer cells. This means the berry extract murdered nine times more cancer cells than the ascorbic solution. You can agree from this study that berries have powerful antioxidizing ability and should help you deal with inflammation-related medical conditions. Lastly, in other studies, berries have been shown to help improve memory in participants showing early signs of memory decline.

Perhaps let me add some more information on the value of fruits in general. As you already know, fruits come in a wide selection including bananas, apples, lemons, mangoes, peaches, oranges, papayas, pineapples, and so on. You are bound to find a fruit you like best. Generally, fruits have high water content, which helps you stay hydrated while containing a low concentration of fat (should help maintain heart health). In Vedic fasting, fruits form part of the meal because they are thought to promote Satwa (restfulness and creativity) in the body. In fruits, you are likely to find mostly sugars (pears contain 6.5% of fructose and 1.3% of sucrose) and fiber which is fermented in the colon to keep the gut clean.

Some fruits like grapefruit have been shown to help with weight loss (your main goal), reduce insulin levels in the bloodstream, and also help lower insulin resistance. Not only that, they help lower cholesterol levels and aid to block the formation of kidney stones. On the other hand, watermelons contain important antioxidants such as lycopene and carotenoids. Lycopene helps reduce cholesterol levels and blood pressure, and thus may improve heart health. The excessive amount of water in a watermelon (92%) helps you become full. Watermelons have been linked with a reduced risk of stomach and intestine problems, while oranges and lemons contain high levels of vitamin C which contain citric acid to help treat kidney stones.

Most importantly, most fruits contain folic acid that helps in formation of red blood cells, the chief ingredient in blood. So, it is vital to add fruits in the meals you eat during the feeding window of your fasting protocol to obtain the necessary nutrients, vitamins and fiber. You can choose any fruit you prefer, but ensure you eat it while it is fresh if you can.

2. Lentils

This food item falls into the legume family and is rich in fiber, carbohydrates and proteins. A single cup of cooked lentils contains 16 grams of fiber essential for proper bowel movement in the digestive tract. The beauty is that lentils can be prepared in a variety of ways such as soup and salad. This nutrient-dense legume is packed with minerals such as magnesium, calcium, potassium, zinc and phosphorus, as well as essential amino acids.

3. Soybeans

This legume food is of East Asian origin and is rich with proteins. The dietary fiber it has makes you feel full and helps to reduce your intake of carbs while slowing down digestion. With an abundant soy protein, this legume has been found to help lower bad cholesterol (LDL) levels, because it has a low saturated fat content. This means soybeans can help lower the risk of heart disease. A review study done in 2015, reported in the *British Journal of Nutrition*, found that intake of soybeans does not only lower LDL cholesterol levels, but it significantly increases the concentration of good HDL cholesterol.

Finally, soybeans are a great source of nutrients and vitamins such as vitamin C, calcium, magnesium, phosphorus, potassium, thiamine, and folate.

4. Nuts

There are a variety of nuts including walnuts, cashews, almonds, and macadamia nuts. Nuts also fall in the legume family and contain high fat content, proteins, carbs, fiber, vitamin E, magnesium, phosphorus, copper, manganese, and selenium.

The fiber they contain is a source of food for microbiota in the large intestine. These gut bacteria ferment the fiber and turn it into short-chain fatty acids that help improve gut health.

A small 2014 study of 16 healthy adults discovered that walnuts help in weight loss and may decrease cholesterol and triglycerides. Another 2013 study of 47 caucasian subjects investigated the impact of a walnut-enriched diet on the burning of lipids and glucose in the body as well as inflammation, adipokines, and endothelial function. The results agreed with the 2014 study and showed a significant drop in non-HDL cholesterol and apolipoprotein-B. Other research has shown that regularly eating walnuts tends to decrease coronary heart disease and helps to reduce blood sugar levels in patients with type 2 diabetes and metabolic syndrome. And lastly, nuts may assist in reducing oxidative stress and blood pressure.

5. Healthy Fats

The most important source of healthy fats is avocados, an important source of healthy monounsaturated fatty acids. Avocados are nutrient-dense and include about 20 vitamins and minerals and the most common of these are vitamins C, E, K, and B1 to B6, plus riboflavin, niacin, folic acid, potassium, magnesium, lutein, beta-carotene and omega-3 fatty acids. Because of the high amount of fats, avocados help you to become satiated and full, inducing the brain to turn off appetite. That means you'll be able to reduce the amount of calories you take in, which will aid with weight loss and lower metabolism of carbohydrates and thus keep blood glucose levels more stable. Healthy fat further promotes skin health, may boost the immune system, and helps to notch-up absorption of fat-soluble vitamins, minerals, and other nutrients.

Here's a summary of what the other minerals help your body to do:

- Beta sitosterol helps stabilize healthy cholesterol levels.
- Phytochemicals (antioxidants) help minimize damage to the eyes, promoting your vision.
- Potassium supports bone health by supporting the absorption of calcium and reducing the amount of calcium excreted through the urine.
- Folate helps lower risk of depression and therefore reduces anxiety, while also helping to prevent an increase in the

concentration of homocysteine that can negatively impact circulation and delivery of nutrients to the energy-intensive brain.

- High amounts of fiber helps to prevent constipation and so, helps to maintain a healthy digestive tube as well as lowering the risk of colon cancer.

- Saponins are associated with relieving the signs of knee osteoarthritis.

6. Fish and Seafood

In general, seafood is pregnant with proteins, vitamin D, zinc, iodine, iron, and omega-3 fatty acids. Salmon has been branded as a superfood, and for good reason. It is a rich source of lean protein and therefore, may help with weight loss. The omega-3 fatty acids help lower the risk of autoimmune ailments. A combination of selenium and vitamin B12 may boost a person's immune system and resist easy attack by bacteria and viruses. In addition, the zinc in salmon, and most other seafoods, helps with cell growth.

Vitamin D and the fatty acids assist with improving bone health, while omega-3 fatty acids have also been specifically associated with lowering the risk of heart attack, diabetes and improving cognitive function.

Seafood is considered a low-calorie food and the protein it has is easier to digest because the flesh is softer than red meat and poultry.

Chapter 7: Seven Extra Benefits of Intermittent Fasting 16/8

There is no doubt that intermittent fasting 16/8 helps with weight loss. Are there other benefits you may get from intermittent fasting? Absolutely. We'll look at a number of benefits that scientific research has proven can accrue for anyone who consistently practices intermittent fasting 16/8. These benefits include protection against deteriorating metabolism and cognitive function, and reversal of type 2 diabetes.

Fasting can Reverse Type 2 Diabetes

In 2019, diabetes was estimated to have been responsible for the death of about 4.2 million people worldwide aged 20 to 79 years. Not only is this story sad, the fact that over 463 million adults live with diabetes is scary. And of these people, 90% have type 2 diabetes.

As you know, there are two kinds of diabetes. Type 1 diabetes occurs when the body is not able to produce its own insulin. Lack of insulin in the body over a long time is not only dangerous, but can lead to damage of key body organs and health complications such as cardiovascular diseases, nerve damage, kidney damage and eye disease. It is this kind of diabetes which can be addressed with insulin injection and other diet strategies. The second kind is called type 2 diabetes. It takes root due to lifestyle and ways of eating. That's why it is seen as a dietary and lifestyle disease. Here is how a person becomes type 2 diabetic.

Most people today eat multiple times during the day. Coupled with snacks, we are almost always eating. As urbanization becomes the norm throughout the world, more people live sedentary lifestyles and consume unhealthy food associated with obesity. Who can blame us with so much abundance of food and easy access to resources? Unfortunately, a continuous supply of food causes a sustained high level of glucose and insulin in the bloodstream. The body cells become saturated with glucose. At the same time, more glucose is stored as glycogen, but the liver can only store so much of it. So, some of the glucose is converted to fat and when this hyperglycaemic condition is maintained for too long, the body adapts and becomes insulin-resistant. And we say the person now has type 2 diabetes. Unfortunately, medication only tries to force more glucose into the cells; it does not deal with the root cause of this diabetes. It is here where intermittent fasting comes in. In fact, *IDF Diabetes Atlas, 9th edition* (2019) makes a statement that sums up how to deal with type 2 diabetes. This is what they say, "The cornerstone of type 2 diabetes management is the promotion of a lifestyle that includes a healthy diet, regular physical activity, smoking cessation and maintenance of a healthy body weight." And intermittent fasting 16/8 is an effective lifestyle to attain and maintain a healthy body weight and therefore manage or even reverse type 2 diabetes.

During fasting, no new glucose enters the body and as such, the body is forced to use glucose already in the bloodstream, the cells, and liver for energy.

Once this glucose is depleted, the body begins to use stored fat as a source of energy. A prolonged fasting program may eventually reset the glucose and insulin levels in the bloodstream and finally reverse the diabetic condition. Type 2 diabetes is often associated with obesity, so reversing this diabetes is often accompanied by loss of weight.

Although we explained it in this simplistic manner, and we must, it is important for any diabetic person to visit their physician before making any change of diet. The reason is for the physician to adjust their medication to match the new diet so intermittent fasting 16/8 becomes safe.

Improvement in Well-being of People with Multiple Sclerosis (MS)

It is estimated that there are about 400,000 U.S. citizens that have multiple sclerosis, while worldwide, the number of such patients is about 2.5 million. Multiple sclerosis is believed to be an autoimmune disease where the immune system gouges the protective layer of nerve fibers. As a result, this chronic illness can result in catastrophic damage of the nerves and may cause disability. A major concern is that it causes miscommunication between the brain and the body. But all is not lost.

Research by Fitzgerald and his colleagues, approved by the Johns Hopkins School of Medicine Institutional Review Board, gives hope that intermittent fasting can reverse the condition. These experts, encouraged by favorable effects of intermittent fasting on mice, wanted to investigate if humans with multiple sclerosis could also benefit. In addition, they also wanted to test if intermittent fasting is safe for people with this challenge. Their secondary intents included checking on intermittent fasting's impact on fatigue, sleep, and mood.

They recruited 36 participants for this 8-week study, but only 31 completed it. Meals were prepared and supplied to the study subjects by the U.S. Department of Agriculture and were tailored to each individual's specific calorie needs. This is important as each person's diet needs differ from that of the next person. Now, what were the results of this trial?

As expected, the subjects lost a weight of between 3.0kg and 3.6kg depending on whether they did alternate day fasting or daily fasting (as suggested in this book). Participants who were on daily calorie restriction, lost more weight than the alternate day fasters. Interestingly, daily fasting had fewer drop-outs than alternate day fasting participants. The researchers further found that the study subjects experienced a significant decline in cholesterol levels. Best of all, the participants' emotional well-being also improved. The major concern participants raised during this investigation was that they battled with hunger, something common to most beginning practitioners of any fasting protocol. Although the study was short, it gave encouraging signs that fasting can help overweight people with multiple sclerosis improve their well-being while losing weight at the same time.

How Fasting Ended Stomach Pain

Once, in ancient Rome, lived a man called Agricola. He was a nephew of the famous poet and statesman, Cicero. Agricola suffered from stomach pains for many years. He had tried many different kinds of medicines with no success at all. Finally, he decided the best cure for him was to die and he chose to fast himself to death. Surprisingly, instead of dying, Agricola unknowingly killed the disease that had abused him for so long. What had happened here?

The answer is simple. You see, during fasting, Agricola had given his hard-working stomach a deserved rest. And nature chipped in and did its magic. So it is with anyone who adopts a fasting lifestyle. Fasting helps clear the stomach of any foreign matter that affects human and even animal health. Have a look at how fasting helped a buffalo calf at the brink of death.

A rich merchant in India had a herd of buffalo. One of the buffalo calves got sick to the point of death.

The merchant, his family, and workers had tried all the tricks in the book to no avail. One day, a younger member of the family thought it was better to just untie the calf and let it die. So, he instructed one of the family helpers to untie the calf. Immediately, the calf trotted to a sunny spot at an open space. It stayed there for a while, then returned to the shade and drank cold water. Then it went back to the sunny area and later returned to the shade and again, drank cold water. It never ate any food. The calf repeated this for three consecutive days. And on the fourth day, the calf got cured from its malady. Indeed, fasting can help cure diseases which at times startle even the most educated doctors.

Fasting Improves Brain Function

It is well-known that the human brain uses about 20% of the energy supplied to the body. It must do so because this organ controls most of the functions of the human body. As such, it is essential to keep it healthy and energized by feeding it essential nutrients. However, it has been established that our cognitive abilities jump up a few notches when we are hungry, that is, we tend to think better on empty stomachs than when we are full.

When we are satiated, more blood flows to the digestive system to supply the needed energy to break down nutrients. This reduces the amount of blood that marches throughout the brain. So, our thinking function tends to decline during this time. No wonder, some of us feel sluggish or even sleepy after having a heavy meal. Fasting, on the other hand, has an opposite effect of improving our brain functioning.

Aging has a tendency to cause a decline in memory, learning and motor control. But all is not lost. A study by Shin and colleagues at Hoseo University was done to establish if intermittent fasting can protect against the declining cognitive function in Alzheimer's disease-induced estrogen-deficient rats. The researchers divided the rats into two groups, with one group following intermittent fasting while the other was fed as and when required. This study discovered, as expected, that Alzheimer's disease impaired cognitive function, disturbed energy, glucose, lipid, and bone metabolism. However, intermittent fasting prevented memory loss and metabolic disturbances. So, intermittent fasting can help you remember facts like people's names, doctor's appointments, and even your child's birthdays. After menopause, women tend to suffer loss of energy, poor glucose and lipids metabolism, and experience cognitive dysfunction, and intermittent fasting can be of immense help here as well.

Numerous other tests done on aging mice showed that a calorie-restricted diet did not show declines in motor coordination and spatial learning. Also, it has been proven that periodic fasting can increase neurogenesis (a process where adult brain cells divide and then differentiate into new neurons). This means through fasting, besides losing weight, you can grow new neurons, which in turn, help with brain functioning.

Research has also shown that intermittent fasting reduces insulin levels in our bloodstream. This is good news for this reason. High insulin can cause a decline in memory and so, reducing insulin favors the improvement in remembering. There are other benefits to fasting.

Fasting Slows Aging

The human body is made up of smaller units called cells. The cell components get damaged and require renewal for the cell to keep living. But renewal of the cell components takes place for a limited time. At some point, cells must be replaced. This is where a process called autophagy comes in. What is autophagy?

Autophagy is a name derived from Greek and it means *eating of self*. Therefore, autophagy is a natural, orderly process for renewing cell components. Our bodies get renewed regularly. Unfortunately, today's ways of eating and lifestyle do not promote this cell-renewing mechanism.

Regular eating maintains high levels of glucose, insulin and proteins in the bloodstream and this inactivates autophagy. This means there will be a build-up of dead cell components in the body and over time, diseases like cancer may occur as does rapid aging. However, there is a way out.

Intermittent fasting helps reduce glucose levels in the blood and subsequently promotes low insulin. When this happens, autophagy is activated and house cleaning begins in earnest. So, practicing long-term intermittent fasting eventually eliminates the potential for some body cells to become cancerous, while at the same time the body gets renewed and delays the aging process. Let's look at some more advantages of intermittent fasting.

Intermittent Fasting Helps Improve Heart Health

Data by the U.S. National Center for Health Statistics revealed that the top cause of death in the

U.S. is heart disease with almost 650,000 casualties. Cancer came second at almost 600,000 deaths. The World Health Organization reports that 31% (17.9 million) of all annual deaths worldwide are due to cardiovascular diseases. These are staggering numbers, aren't they? Sure, they are. To make the situation even more dire, 33% of these deaths happen to people below the age of 70 years who still have so much to give to the world. Unfortunately, life robs us of their valued contribution. To add insult to injury, 80% of deaths from cardiovascular diseases occur as a result of heart attacks and stroke. You'll agree this situation calls for an effective, yet easy to apply, remedy.

As you know, heart attacks and stroke are often the result of poor health and it has been established that high-risk people tend to have high blood pressure, high blood sugar levels, and lipids, and are overweight and obese.

Numerous studies have attempted to figure out what the impact of intermittent fasting is to cardiovascular diseases. And indeed, intermittent fasting was found to improve risk factors such as high blood pressure, high sugar levels, total and LDL cholesterol, and blood triglycerides. For example, a 2009 research study focused on the effect of intermittent fasting on weight loss and heart protection in obese adults. The study recruited 12 women and four men for the 10-week trial. Encouragingly, these people succeeded in losing weight and best of all, total cholesterol, lDL cholesterol, and systolic blood pressure decreased.

Another study investigated the impact of intermittent fasting on cardiovascular stress on rats. The researchers induced cardiovascular stress on these rats and then took their subjects through intermittent fasting. Results showed the rats rapidly returned to their normal blood pressures and heart rates. These are encouraging signs indeed for people who may be overweight or obese.

Intermittent Fasting May Reduce Inflammation in the Body

Normally, inflammation is the mechanism that the body uses to respond to injuries by healing itself or to fight invaders like germs, chemicals, and injuries. However, chronic inflammation has been linked as one of the causes of certain chronic illnesses like heart diseases, rheumatoid arthritis (where many joints throughout the body are permanently inflamed), psoriasis, and even skin disorders like eczema. If you get a small cut on your finger, for example, your body immediately releases hormones that dilate the small blood vessels to allow more blood to flow to the affected area. This blood carries with it more immune system cells to the injured spot to heal it.

Inflammation has also been associated with a condition known as leptin resistance. If there's a low concentration of leptin in the blood, the brain activates your appetite so that you can eat. Once you have eaten, your fat stores increase. On the other hand, if there are high levels of leptin in the blood, the reverse happens. The brain suppresses your appetite and then you feel like not eating.

In certain cases, the brain is not able to receive messages whether there's low or high leptin in the blood. This condition is called leptin resistance. The brain and the body are always concerned about our safety. So, when something is not right within the body, they initiate a safety-first approach. When the body is in leptin-resistance mode, the brain activates your appetite because it assumes there isn't sufficient leptin in the bloodstream. As a result, your appetite is almost always on. This means you'll eat often and force your body to store a lot of fat in the fat cells. And thus, you may become and stay overweight and even obese. The first, and perhaps most important step, is to get your leptin levels tested. In fasting mode, your leptin levels typically range from 4 to 6 nanograms per decilitre of blood. If you get higher numbers, that's a sign you may be leptin resistant. Now, how do you deal with inflammation? Intermittent fasting has been shown to help the body reduce inflammation.

Take for example an 8-week study conducted by J. B. Johnson of the Department of Surgery, Louisiana State University Medical Center, New Orleans, and his colleagues, reported in *Free Radical Biology and Medicine* journal. These researchers were curious to find out what effect intermittent fasting has on indicators of oxidative stress and inflammation in overweight, asthmatic patients. At the start, and at selected time intervals, our experts assessed and collected blood samples to analyze for general health, asthma control, and symptoms, as well as oxidative stress plus inflammation. In just two weeks, asthma-related symptoms improved significantly and stayed that way throughout the research. Excitingly, these experts discovered remarkable reductions in markers of oxidative stress such as protein carbonyls and improved concentrations of uric acid, an antioxidant. Inflammation markers like brain-derived neurotrophic factor decreased significantly. This is how the researchers concluded their eye-opening research,

"Compliance with the ADCR diet was high, symptoms and pulmonary function improved, and oxidative stress and inflammation declined in response to the dietary intervention." (Johnson et al, p. 665–674, 2007). There you have it.

The foregoing clearly shows there's more to gain from intermittent fasting 16/8 than just losing weight. Your overall health receives a boost and you are able to fight off major concerns as stated above.

Now, you may still be unconvinced that intermittent fasting 16/8 is a safe and effective way to shed excess weight. I don't know what your biggest concern may be, but below, I answer several common concerns about intermittent fasting.

Chapter 8: Ten Common Concerns Fasters Have and How to Handle Them

At this point, you are probably wondering if intermittent fasting 16/8 is a perfect way to lose weight and gain energy. The biggest doubt, perhaps, is whether we have not hidden any side-effects that may hurt you if you adopt this weight loss protocol. Look, intermittent fasting 16/8 is not a perfect, holy grail of weight loss. There are some challenges you may encounter as you fast, especially at the beginning. As you know, habits die hard. The mind and body don't become quickly accustomed to a new way of living instantaneously. They tend to change following a gradual adjustment process.

In intermittent fasting 16/8, there are some concerns you may have and we would like to address them right now. You may have heard that intermittent fasting can cause things like headaches, hair loss, fatigue, muscle loss, gastritis, bloating, and so on. Let's now address some of these concerns.

Why Am I not Losing Weight on Intermittent Fasting 16/8

This is probably one of the biggest concerns people who want to lose weight may face. I want to caution you upfront about weight loss. If you look closely at what happens within your body, you'll notice that a lot of change occurs. The heart rate is a good example. It always goes up and down, which means you cannot target a specific heart rate. But you can target a heart rate of between 65 and 90 beats per minute as the ideal. So it is with weight loss. Your ideal weight will fluctuate from a certain low to a specific high. Hence, don't expect your weight to stay at a constant value. That will just be inviting unwanted stress. With that out of the way, it is now time to go over several reasons why you may not lose weight during intermittent fasting.

You May be Consuming Excessive Carbohydrates than Your Body Requires

We shared two recent research studies that concluded that there's no common diet for everyone. This means as an intermittent faster, you have a unique diet that is suitable for your body and lifestyle. For this reason, your first step is to discover what that diet is, that is, how many macros of carbs, proteins and fat are suitable for your body to enter into ketosis each time you fast.

The starting point is to figure out your carb tolerance level. Carb tolerance level means the maximum amount of carbs your body can take and still enter ketosis during fasting. This is how to go about it:

- Start consuming your carbs where they currently are.
- Measure your ketone levels, preferably blood ketones, after 12 hours of fasting. Also measure your glucose levels.

- You must be in ketosis by then. If not, it is a sign you must reduce the amount of carbs you consume at dinner (if your fast begins after dinner, that is) until you enter into ketosis after 12 hours of fasting.
- If you are in ketosis, great.

Note: This procedure assumes you are eating a moderate amount of proteins, about 15% to 20% of your daily calorie intake.

There's another reason why you may be consuming too much carbs. It is that you may be missing some hidden carbs in your meals. There are carbs in foods like cabbage and cauliflower. If you are not careful, you can quickly consume a sizable amount of carbs from them without knowing. So, be on the lookout for such kinds of food.

You May be Consuming Excessive Proteins

The body is an efficient machine. It does not waste time and energy doing work that is not essential. It is designed to be able to convert proteins into glucose via a process called gluconeogenesis, as we said earlier. This process follows immediately when stored glucose (called glycogen) is depleted. This is the time when the body turns to proteins to convert them into glucose.

What you want is that this glucose from proteins should be inadequate for the body's energy requirements. This would force the body to use stored fat as an energy source. It is essential, therefore, to supply the body with enough proteins while still getting into ketosis. And thus, you must determine your body's protein tolerance level. Here's how to go about it:

- Measure ketone bodies in your blood after 12 hours of fasting.
- If you notice no ketones in blood, reduce your protein intake in your next meal. Then, measure ketones after the next fast to check if you are in ketosis.
- Repeat this process until you see ketones in your blood.

We assume that you are changing the amount of proteins while keeping your carbs more or less the same.

There's an interesting research study that was done by Fromentin of the National Institute for Agronomic Research, Ile-de-France Human Nutrition Research Center, and colleagues titled, "Dietary Proteins Contribute Little to Glucose Production, Even Under Optimal Gluconeogenic Conditions in Healthy Humans." (Fromentin et al, 2012, p. 1435–1442). What this study found was that most of the proteins we consume are not immediately used for much of gluconeogenesis.

What the researchers did was give 8 participants, who had fasted throughout the night, glucose first thing in the morning. Two hours later, they gave the participants four eggs. Finally, they tracked gas exchanges, expired carbon dioxide, blood, and urine for eight hours.

What they discovered was that only about 18% of the dietary proteins participated in gluconeogenesis. This is fascinating. It suggests that during gluconeogenesis, the body tends to prefer to use proteins already stored in the body for gluconeogenesis. It is therefore essential to determine your protein tolerance level as suggested above.

You May be Having Leptin Resistance

Leptin is a hormone that regulates and controls appetite in humans. It gets instructions from the hypothalamus area (a part of the brain) that includes the hippocampus. This part of the brain is responsible not only to control and regulate appetite, but to also regulate and control growth and reproduction.

Leptin is produced in the fat cells, kidneys, salivary glands, and stomach. Once produced, it enters the bloodstream. This blood flow nourishes all parts of the body, including the brain. So, leptin's concentration in the blood tells the brain whether to tell you to eat or not. In other words, leptin plays a significant role in hunger control.

It is a good move to check leptin concentration in your blood if you suspect you may be leptin-resistant. The major cause of leptin resistance is a condition called inflammation. Fortunately, there is a way to fight inflammation. It responds to certain foods like healthy fats, fish and nuts when they form part of your diet. You would do well to minimize eating too much in the way of saturated fats.

The other thing to do is to lower your stress levels because it may attack leptin receptors in your brain and thus block leptin messages from reaching the brain's leptin control center.

You May be Doing Too Little or Excessive Physical Activity

Any diet depends on the energy balance of the body for its effectiveness. Energy balance is the difference in energy between energy intake and energy expenditure. When energy intake far exceeds energy expenditure, the body is forced to store some for future use. It stores the energy in the form of glycogen and fat. This is what too little exercise makes the body do. Hence, the person may become overweight or even obese.

Physical activity does not necessarily mean hitting the gym or running on the road every morning and evening. No. It means doing some physical activities like walking, cutting a tree, doing a bit of gardening, cooking, cleaning, walking up and down the stairs at work, chopping wood, and so on. Doing these activities requires more energy than when seated in front of a television or a cinema screen.

On the other hand, too much physical activity can get your appetite juices into full gear. If you have a weak willpower, the appetite will win the battle. And thus, you may eat a lot more and your body will keep burning carbs instead of fat. You want your body to burn fat during fasting as soon as you begin the fast.

You May be Having Inadequate Sleep.

Modern day life is very busy. Night has become like day. The activities that used to be done only in the day are easily done during the night, including things like shopping. We also watch television countless hours per day. It's common knowledge that North Americans watch about seven hours of television per day on average. That's almost 30% of a day. All this is made possible by advances in technology.

Unfortunately, this comes at a cost because the amount of sleeping time is reduced. Less sleep has been proven to affect the energy expenditure of a person. A study by Nedeltcheva, of the Department of Medicine, University of Chicago, and colleagues in 2010 called "Insufficient sleep undermines dietary efforts to reduce adiposity" discovered interesting facts about how sleep affects us. Here's what the researchers did. They recruited 12 participants aged between 35 and 49. These people normally slept for between 6.5 hours and 8.5 hours per day. All were healthy. The study took place from July 2003 to July 2008. The participants then spent two 14-day periods in a laboratory environment where they were allowed to sleep for 8.5 hours or 5.5 hours per night in random order.

Researchers gave each participant the same kind of meal as the others during the 14 days. The calories in the meals were restricted to 90% of that required by the body during rest. This meal condition mimicked what people tend to do when they go on diets or intermittent fasting. What they discovered was that less sleep with reduced calorie intake decreases loss of fat when compared to sleeping 8.5 hours. They also found that the less-sleepers, if I may call them that, had increased loss of fat-free mass.

The logical explanation is that insufficient sleep makes the body prefer fat-free macronutrients stored in the body for energy. The most likely macronutrient burnt this way is proteins. This research suggests that when you are fasting, it's essential to have sufficient sleep (your body will let you know this) during each day as far as possible.

You May be Experiencing Too Much Stress.

When the mind is under stress, the brain releases a hormone known as cortisol into the bloodstream. This hormone is also found in hair. Yes, hair. An extensive study of 2 527 English men and women made astonishing discoveries. The researchers believed chronic cortisol levels contributed to obesity. So, they went ahead to prove or disprove their educated guess (a hypothesis).

The study made this statement about the findings, "In cross-sectional analyses, hair cortisol concentrations were positively correlated with body weight, BMI (body mass index), and waist circumference, and were significantly elevated in participants with obesity and raised waist circumference." The researchers also discovered that high hair cortisol levels persisted for over four years for the participants who were obese.

It's pretty clear that stress therefore affects body weight. The reason has to do with the tendency some people have to eat more in volume and more often when they are stressed. Of course, more food means more calories and the body has no choice but to store some of this as fat. Much more importantly, cortisol affects not only the quantity but also the type of food we consume. It must be for this reason that junk food flies off the shelves in today's stressful lives.

How do you deal with stress? In two ways. The obvious thing to do is to avoid stress-causing physical and psychological events. But this is not always easy because some events may be out of your control. For example, you may be stressed because a fire licked your whole house because of an electric fault. You had little to do with this. But it can affect your brain functioning. But there are other things you can control.

For example, you can control what you think about an event that has occurred. This is possible since you were born with the ability to control your thoughts. Unfortunately, most of us were not trained to do this. And we feel like it's impossible to direct our thoughts. Just as an example. A man called Viktor Frankl, who was a Jewish psychiatrist, explains in his book, *Man's Search for Meaning*, how he did that when he was in Hitler's concentration camp. In fact, it was during this time that he discovered that controlling your thoughts is really the only freedom that you can ever have on this beautiful planet earth. This is what is called responding as opposed to reacting.

So, make the choice today to respond to events rather than only react like the majority of people do.

Failure to Adapt to Intermittent Fasting 16/8

A diet tweak normally stresses the body and the brain. The latter in turn instructs the body to release this stress by indulging in the old diet. Unfortunately, doing this will certainly prevent you from achieving your fasting goals.

It is during this adaptive stage to your new eating pattern that you may face the most challenges. This is the time when your resolve will be tested. You'll find yourself wondering whether going on a fast was the right decision or not. Let me assure you, it was the right decision, only that the body is now adapting to a new way of eating. Remember we said earlier that we are creatures of habit? It is like going to a gym for the first time. The following day, the body usually aches to show you it didn't like what you did. But if you want the benefits that come with physical exercise, what do you do? Of course, you go back to the gym again and again and again. Why? Because from resistance comes strength. Eventually, the pain goes away and you begin to enjoy your gym exercises.

So it is with intermittent fasting 16/8. In the beginning, the body will certainly revolt. Your only recourse is to remind yourself why you made the choice to go on intermittent fasting in the first place. Read the little piece of paper we spoke about in the first chapter to remind yourself of this important decision. Then, recommit to your weight loss goal.

I'm reminded here about what Robin Sharma, the author of the famed *The Monk Who Sold His Ferrari*, once said. He put it better than I could when he said, "All change is hard at first, messy in the middle and gorgeous in the end." Isn't that great? I certainly agree with him and I hope you do as well.

Adapting to intermittent fasting takes varying durations for different people. For some, it can be a few weeks and others, a few months. The key is to adjust your diet as we suggested earlier on determining your carb and protein tolerances. These measurements will guide you to make informed decisions, unlike making blind decisions.

Your main challenges during this adapting stage will be conditions such as nausea, vomiting, headache, dizziness, fatigue, constipation, and difficulty in exercising. We discuss some of these challenges below.

It's unusual for one person to experience all these symptoms at the same time. If you do experience any of them, take in adequate fluids and electrolytes. The minerals contained in these fluids will influence your blood chemistry and alter the body. However, you should now remind yourself that this is only a transition to the promised land, the weight you've always dreamt about.

You May be Drinking Alcohol Containing Too Many Carbs

Beverages like beer contain appreciable amounts of carbs. They, therefore, can increase the amount of carbs to beyond your tolerance level. Better take the hard alcoholic stuff like vodka, whisky, brandy, and tequila which have low carbs in them.

Does Intermittent Fasting 16/8 Cause Hair Loss?

Hair loss is a common concern with about 50% of men and women affected by the time they hit the 50-year mark. Let's get the scientific facts right away. Hair growth is affected by a number of factors including calorie deficiency, lack of proteins, and micronutrients such as Vitamin A, selenium, and Vitamin E in the body. This may also affect hair structure and hair growth. Over-supplementation of selenium, Vitamin A and Vitamin E may also have an impact on hair loss. Other nutrients found to impact hair growth and structure include zinc and iron.

Iron deficiency: It is known that iron is one of the nutrients lacking in human nutrition. Further, iron deficiency is a big role-player in hair loss. However, how the mechanism involved isn't clear.

Zinc deficiency: Scientists know zinc is essential in the working of several enzymes. Just like with iron, the exact way it gets involved in the enzymes that affect gene expression is not known. These experts, however, believe zinc influences the Hedgehog signaling pathway, one of the key components that controls hair follicle morphogenesis. In a research study of 312 participants with male pattern hair loss, it was found that the patients had lower zinc concentration than 30 healthy patients in the control group.

Deficiency of the fatty acid linoleic acid: This can occur as a result of inappropriate nutrition and has been linked with scalp hair loss and eyebrows.

So, intermittent fasting by itself does not cause hair loss. The reason is because this fasting regime still allows you to eat and get the necessary nutrients into your body. What is key, however, is the type of food you eat. As we suggested above, it is important to eat nutrient-dense meals during the feeding cycle so you stay healthy.

Does Intermittent Fasting 16/8 Cause Gastritis?

A practitioner of intermittent fasting said something which this book must answer or else false information will keep making the rounds, and stop most people from benefiting via intermittent fasting 16/8. This faster said his doctor told him that going 18 hours without eating might attack the internal lining of the stomach due to gastric juices released during mid-day. I wonder if the doctor has any idea how digestion occurs. Anyway, let me plainly reveal the facts.

What is gastritis? In short, it is the inflammation of the internal lining of the stomach. Its main cause is a bacterium known as Helicobacter pylori, which attacks the stomach lining. This germ is commonly transmitted by infected food or water. Other major causes include:

- Smoking.
- Aging: The stomach lining may become thinner due to normal wear and tear.
- Drinking excessive alcohol.
- Regular use of medication such as aspirin and ibuprofen.

Now, and this is important, the stomach releases gastric juices when stimulated by food. During the abstaining period of intermittent fasting 16/8, the only processes taking place are digestion and elimination of chyme into the small intestine. Clearly, there's no factual way intermittent fasting can cause gastritis. However, it is important to keep hydrated to encourage cleaning of the stomach. And fasting should help clear any gastritis-causing agents out of the stomach because it is an efficient house-cleaning mechanism of the digestive tract.

Intermittent Fasting 16/8 and Bloating

Bloating occurs when ingested food is digested poorly. This food then ferments and causes gas, which tends to fill the digestive tract (stomach and the intestines). When in this condition, you'll normally experience stomach rumblings as the gas passes from one region of the digestive tube to another. Poor digestion tends to occur mostly in nervous fasters and may cause pain, while in relaxed fasters this is unlikely. In the event there is gas in the stomach, it usually is in small quantities to cause discomfort. But for some fasters this gas may be enough to cause distress and sleeplessness. Fasters with a history of issues are top candidates for internal tensions of the digestive tract.

The way to address the bloating challenge is to relax, which should relieve nervousness and internal tension. Drinking water is important as it may aid in proper digestion. Importantly, when experiencing bloating, continue to fast as this gives your digestive system rest and fights with the bloat. To supplement these efforts, during your feeding period, eat easily digestible food such as cooked spinach and zucchini.

Can Intermittent Fasting 16/8 Cause Muscle Loss?

Typically, when an intermittent faster loses weight, the bulk of the flesh removed is visceral fat, while subcutaneous fat and lean mass are spared. But is that fact? Let's set our opinions aside and visit the pages of science for evidence.

A study in 2016, reported in *Obesity*, was conducted to find out if alternate-day fasting (ADF) is safe and tolerable. The secondary intents included comparing alternate-day fasting with a calorie-restricted weight loss protocol. What the researchers did was recruit obese participants aged from 18 to 55 years for this 8-week test at the University of Colorado. All the participants underwent a thorough medical history and physical exam, including measurements of uric acid, blood pressure, heart rate, and liver functions. Of the original participants, 26 completed the 8-week exercise, while 21 finished the 24-week follow-up to check for level of weight gain.

After 8 weeks, these learned researchers found that the participants who were on the alternate-day fasting lost about 1.1 kg more weight than the calorie-restricted group. But there was no difference in the amount of fat lost by both groups of dieters. Most importantly, the study discovered there was no significant difference in lost fat between the two groups. In their words, this is what they said, "There were no significant differences in change in absolute (kg) or relative (%) FM, trunk FM, and LM over the 8-week intervention." Note that FM stands for fat mass and LM for lean mass.

A second study released in *Obesity* in 2010, found that alternate-day fasting does not cause a reduction in fat-free mass, but significantly reduces waist circumference (visceral fat). Here are some of the results from this research:

	Baseline control phase		Weight loss/ADF controlled feeding phase		Weight loss/ feedi
	Day 1	Day 14	Day 41 Feed day	Day 42 Fast day	Day 69 Feed day
Body weight (kg)	96.4 ± 5.3	96.5 ± 5.2	93.8 ± 5.0*	93.7 ± 5.0*	92.8 ± 4.8*
BMI (kg/m²)	33.7 ± 1.0	33.7 ± 1.0	32.8 ± 1.0	32.8 ± 0.9	32.1 ± 0.8*
Fat mass (kg)	43.0 ± 2.2	43.5 ± 2.5	41.8 ± 2.7	41.3 ± 2.7	38.1 ± 2.6*
Fat-free mass (kg)	52.0 ± 3.6	51.4 ± 3.4	51.8 ± 3.8	51.1 ± 3.2	52.8 ± 3.3
Waist circumference (cm)	109 ± 2	109 ± 3	106 ± 3	106 ± 3	105 ± 3*

All values are mean ± s.e.m. Body weight and body composition variables did not change during the baseline period (day 1–14).
*Significantly different from baseline (day 14), P < 0.05 (one-factor ANOVA with Bonferroni analysis).

Figure 7: Baseline and followup body composition
measurements

The conclusion is that intermittent fasting, as well as calorie-restricted diet can cause insignificant muscle loss in some cases, and not in others. This may suggest the importance of getting your body composition measured as you start with intermittent fasting 16/8 and thereafter at regular intervals like monthly. Doing this will allow you to track how your fat-free mass changes and if need be, to make timely adjustments to your meals and/or fasting schedule.

Intermittent Fasting and Bad Breath

Imagine you walked into a social gathering such as a farewell party of one of your work colleagues. The place is packed, and conversations are happening all over the place. Because it is noisy, you have to speak with your friend at close range. As you do, you realize your friend is trying to move his sensitive noise as far from your mouth as he possibly can. Wouldn't you wonder why she behaves that way? Sure, you would. And you'll begin to be self-conscious, won't you? That's what bad breath could do. But, does intermittent fasting cause bad breath?

Despite the fact that there are many causes, intermittent fasting can cause bad breath. The kind of smell is of a fruity alcohol which others describe as metallic. The reason for the smell is because during fasting, as we said in chapter 2, the body burns fat for fuel. And that process produces ketones, responsible for the unpleasant smell. Besides ketosis, dehydration may be a factor during intermittent fasting. When there is no saliva in the mouth, the fluids may be off the correct pH. This tends to encourage bacteria to breed and ferment the food particles that may be lodged in crevices found between the teeth.

So, to manage this bad breath, do the following. Keep hydrated to avoid breeding of bacteria in the mouth in order to maintain the saliva pH at the right level. Most importantly, thoroughly brush and floss your teeth to remove any hidden food remains in your mouth.

Can Intermittent Fasting 16/8 Cause Headaches?

Let me not beat about the bush and be straight with you. Intermittent fasting 16/8 may cause headaches. But the headaches come because the body is responding to a loss of the kind of habits it is used to. For example, your fasting protocol may involve withdrawing from things such as tobacco, coffee, tea, drugs, and other stimulants of the nervous system. The body, as we have said before, hates change, especially sudden change.

Quick change usually puts the body and mind in distress as the hormone cortisol begins to concentrate in the bloodstream. This hormone is known to increase appetite so the body can build fat reserves. So, when you stop drinking coffee, for example, cortisol wants you to continue taking this caffeine-containing beverage and it instructs the brain to let you know. If you relent and drink the coffee, you will be astonished how quickly the headache disappears. Never give in to these headache symptoms as their intention is for you to stay overweight and sluggish. I know that's not what you want.

The other cause of headaches during intermittent fasting 16/8 may be due to low blood glucose levels. As you know already, fasting tends to reduce blood glucose levels and insulin levels to favor burning of fat. In some cases, blood sugar may be abnormally low. Now, insufficient glucose will reach the brain cells, which in turn, will activate hormones like cortisol and ghrelin to trigger appetite so as to restore normal blood sugar levels. As such, you may experience a headache.

Intermittent Fasting and Diarrhea

I came across a story about an intermittent faster that I believe will interest you. This faster had eaten her last meal on a certain day at 18:00 and fasted until the following day at 11:00. Her meal consisted of olive salad, roasted chicken breast on a cheese sauce and onions, a cucumber and tomato. In as little as 30 minutes' time, she felt a strong urge to visit the restroom. Fortunately, she was at home and avoided the embarrassment of what was to come. To her astonishment, she excreted a watery stool. Sadly, this happened every day and she came to expect it. What could have happened here? Was this watery stool triggered by intermittent fasting? You wouldn't want to have this happen to you while at work or with friends at a social gathering, would you? Of course not. Let's visit the facts we know about diarrhea and intermittent fasting and clear the air, plus guide you on how to deal with the situation if it ever happens to you.

You see, there are many causes of diarrhea. Before we jump to them, it's essential to define diarrhea so we are on the same page. Diarrhea is a process where food and nutrients accelerate rapidly through the digestive tract without allowing time for absorption into the bloodstream. What causes indigestion, then?

- The kind of diet you consume may cause indigestion. If your meal lacks fiber (from vegetables and fruits), food moves faster through the digestive tube.
- Hormonal changes. A change in hormones may cause the digestive tract to react and induce diarrhea to clean the body.

- Bacteria and parasites. Water or food contaminated with these germs may cause diarrhea.

- Certain medications. A very good example is antibiotics, which can destroy both the good and bad bacteria resulting in a bacterial imbalance in the stomach. This may force rapid bowel removal through the digestive tract, side-stepping adequate intestinal absorption.

- High caffeine consumption. It may trigger the oversecretion of water and salts in the digestive system and the body will react to restore balance.

Intermittent fasting 16/8 is not necessarily the cause of diarrhea. The majority of the time, diarrhea occurs when breaking the fast. As you already know, intermittent fasting puts the digestive system to rest. That slows down bowel movement and fasters usually visit the restroom fewer times than when eating those multiple meals everyday. So, it is essential how and what you eat when you break the fast. It is especially critical to introduce fiber in your meals to help strengthen the waste.

Intermittent Fasting 16/8 and Insomnia

What is insomnia anyway? Insomnia is really the difficulty of falling asleep or staying asleep even when you have the opportunity to do so. When experiencing insomnia, you are likely to feel fatigued, low energy, low concentration, disturbances in mood, and poor performance in what you do like work or studying. Now that we are on the same page on what insomnia is, let's proceed to look if intermittent fasting causes it.

Perhaps this story illustrates some concerns interested fasters may have about intermittent fasting causing insomnia. Let's listen in on this fascinating tale before we delve into what science says about matters like this.

"Yesterday, I began a new dieting protocol called intermittent fasting. So, I ate only one meal all day.

To my surprise, my day went pretty well. For example, I studied tons of material, participated in sports, and completed a number of programming exercises given at the university. After playing some sports, I ate my first meal of the day. In a nutshell, I had a great day with no side-effects from my fasting program. My problems began at 23:00, my bedtime. I could not fall asleep, even for a second. I decided to read a book and an hour went by and I still felt energized. No fatigue at all. I thought doing a few pushups would tire me to no avail. The clock was reading 1:00 a.m. and I had to wake up early. I then tried a glass of brandy and found no happiness. Whatever I tried did not help get me to sleep. So, I finally decided from 4:00 a.m. to just get up and study."

This story reads like a fairy tale, almost unbelievable. It's clearly a story that does tell about insomnia because he had bountiful energy and ability to intensely concentrate. An insomniac would find it hard to read a book for an hour.

It is known that eating times may interfere with the circadian rhythm and impact sleep. All cells in our bodies have circadian clocks. The central clock is housed in the brain area called the hypothalamus. This system requires repetitive calibration and changing the habitual time of taking meals may affect the circadian clock of the body.

Research into whether intermittent fasting causes insomnia is not much. One of the review studies available looked at the impact of diurnal (daytime) intermittent fasting on sleep, daytime sleepiness, and markers of the biological clock. Participants were Ramadan fasters. The research reveals that Ramadan diurnal intermittent fasters experienced a delay in bedtime and wake up time. However, the study could not conclude if the change in the times were due to lifestyle changes during Ramadan or not. Interestingly, this study also discovered that some Ramadan fasters also had delays in bedtime for non-fasters. So, it is inconclusive if intermittent fasting causes insomnia.

Do you remember we said in chapter 4 that people can respond differently to the same meal? If you look closely at people, you'll observe we tend to respond differently to the same things. I'm not surprised when Roger Williams, in his book *Biochemical Individuality* said, "Practically every human being is a deviant in some respects." Our intermittent faster above, who battled with sleep, may have been experiencing his individuality.

Can I Use Intermittent Fasting to Lose Weight when I Have Diabetes?

The story of this 38-year-old obese woman, with type 2 diabetes, serves as a good case to use to answer this question. One time, this lady visited a clinic for her normal diabetes followup. She had been a type 2 diabetic for 6 years. While at the clinic, she told the physician that she craved to lose weight, take less medication and better control her ailment. Her medication included 1000 mg of metformin twice a day, 5 mg of glipizide (a type of sulfonylurea) also two times a day, 40 mg of atorvastatin for hyperlipidemia once a day and 20 mg of lisinopril for hypertension daily.

The woman wanted to know from the physician if she could safely practice intermittent fasting.

Several research studies have proven that intermittent fasting helps with weight loss and improves insulin sensitivity. However, there is fear whether a type 2 diabetic can safely benefit from intermittent fasting. Let's dive into science-backed information to address this concern.

Researchers at Samson Institute of Health Research of the University of South Australia put together a study to find out how intermittent fasting compares with a calorie-restricted meal plan on blood glucose control in patients with type 2 diabetes. To ensure the safety of the patients, researchers were savvy enough to involve the services of a dietician, endocrinologist and the participant's medical practitioners. The main reason for this was because the biggest risk involved with fasting type 2 diabetics is hypoglycemia (excessive low blood glucose levels). And this strategy came in handy when participant 38 entered into a hypoglycemic condition. Immediately, the medical experts adjusted the participant's medications and after 3 months, the researchers never saw a case like that again throughout the 12-month study.

This Australian study made an important and far-reaching observation when it found that, "Intermittent energy restriction is safe for people who have either diet-controlled type 2 diabetes or are using medication that is not likely to cause hypoglycemia. For people using sulfonylureas and/or insulin, intermittent energy restriction requires medication changes and regular monitoring, especially in the initial stages. Patients need to be able to contact their medical practitioner for further medication changes if they experience a hypoglycemic event."

We must agree that it is safe to practice intermittent fasting even if you are diabetic, especially type 2 diabetes. Most importantly, it is essential to involve your physician or medical practitioner before beginning with your intermittent fasting program.

Conclusion: So, What?

You have now reached the end of Intermittent Fasting 16/8 and I applaud you for taking your time to get the right information to lose weight safely and keep it off permanently. It is the first indication that you are serious about losing weight and becoming as energetic as a healthy child. If you have not yet started with intermittent fasting 16/8, you may be wondering what to do next. Wonder no more because I'll provide you with a summary of important ideas and actions to keep in mind for successful weight loss with intermittent fasting 16/8.

Important Steps to Do Right Now

- Decide how much you want to weigh once you are finished with the weight loss process. Note it on a piece of paper like this, "I'm glad now that I weigh between 120 pounds and 130 pounds and I feel great." You choose a range because weight, like any other natural thing, does not stay the same as life progresses.

- Commit to your decision. Remember the little paper I asked you to write in chapter 3? Yes, that one. Read that little document at least once in the morning, once in the afternoon and just before you sleep. Doing this exercise will help you embed your weight loss dream into the subconscious level of your mind where it will be acted on without your constant vigilance.

- Most importantly, before beginning with intermittent fasting 16/8 ensure you take baseline measurements such as blood pressure, fat mass, fat-free mass, insulin levels, waistline circumference and blood glucose levels.

- Now, burn it into your mind that to lose weight permanently, you've got to pay the price. There's nothing called a free lunch. Not paying the price is actually fighting the rules of nature. Any species that did not pay the price immediately perished from the face of the earth. That's how uncompromising nature is. To reap the promised and immense benefits of intermittent fasting 16/8, commit to paying a price equal to gains you want.

Ok. This should be enough to get you started the right way and to build a strong foundation to keep your weight off after losing fat. Now, let me give you a few pointers from the book which you can quickly refer to when necessary.

Takeaways from Chapter 1

- There are two types of hunger; psychological and homeostasis. Psychological hunger drives binge eating, while homeostasis hunger is really hunger that occurs when the body needs refueling.
- Leptin and ghrelin hormones are the main body chemicals that incite appetite and hunger pangs.

- The body requires food so it can get nutrients to burn for energy and to maintain optimal conditions for health.
- Food must be digested before it can be available to the body.
- Digestion occurs in the mouth, stomach, small intestine, and large intestine. Most of the digestion occurs in the small intestine.
- The body burns carbohydrates as the main source of energy.

Takeaways from Chapter 2

- Fasting has been around for thousands of years. People fast for various reasons including political, health, and religious purposes.
- Intermittent fasting 16/8 is a method of fasting for 16 hours and eating during an 8-hour window. It's still important to eat the right kind and amount of food. The main purpose of intermittent fasting 16/8 is to

induce you to take in fewer calories than you normally do.

- When you're fasting, the body turns to fat for energy instead of carbohydrates. Metabolism of fat produces ketones, which can be found in blood, urine or breath. So, measuring ketones is a positive indication of a body that's burning fat. There are devices like breath meters and urine strips you can use to measure ketones.
- Ketoacidosis occurs only when the blood glucose is high and ketone concentration is also high.

Takeaways from Chapter 3

- Most people change eating patterns to lose weight. Yet, many diets don't work.
- The mind is the root cause of failure to lose weight.
- The best way to get the mind to work for you to lose weight is to change the image you have of yourself. See yourself as you want to

be after you've lost the weight. Write a description of this image on a piece of paper and read it often, including in the morning, afternoon and evening before you sleep.

- The subconscious level of your mind houses habits. Any permanent change must change these subconscious habits for lasting results.

Takeaways from Chapter 4

- No two people respond the same way to identical meals. So, you are unique and you must determine the kind of meals that respond positively to your body make-up and lifestyle.
- There are many factors that affect your response to food, including gut microbiota, genetic factors, insulin sensitivity, and so on.

Takeaways from Chapter 5

- The following people should not fast as it is unsafe for them:
    - People under the age of 18.
    - Women who are pregnant or breastfeeding. However, a breastfeeding woman may put the child on baby formula if she must fast.
    - Those having eating disorders such as anorexia.
    - If you have less than 4% body fat.
- If you have gout, diabetes, or are taking medications, ensure you consult your physician before beginning with an intermittent fasting 16/8 program.
- Start by fasting for 12 hours on the first day, then 13 hours the next day, and so on until you hit 16 hours of fasting.
- Small changes make it easy to make bigger changes because the brain accepts them

more readily than big changes to be made in a short time.

- As you fast, you may develop withdrawal symptoms like nausea, vomiting, bad breath, dizziness, headaches, insomnia and others. Continuously remind yourself why you chose to fast so as to persevere over this challenging period. Eventually, these symptoms disappear and you'll enjoy a great intermittent fasting program thereafter.

- Most importantly, take enough water during fasting to stay hydrated and thwart hunger pangs or the urge to snack.

Takeaways from Chapter 6

- Your meals should contain carbohydrates, proteins and fat.

- Berries, like many fruits, are rich in fiber, vitamins, minerals, flavonoids and antioxidants. For this reason, berries help with bowel movement, brain function, and assists with fighting inflammation. They may also help with the clotting of blood and reducing the risk of heart disease and stroke as well the risk of developing kidney stones.

- Eat fresh fruits to avoid consuming added sugar (like that found in bottled juices, for example).

- Some fruits such as grapefruit have shown to help with weight loss.

- Lentils are a nutrient-dense legume rich in proteins, fiber, essential minerals, and carbohydrates.

- Soybeans are a great source of nutrients and vitamins such as vitamin C, calcium, magnesium, phosphorus, potassium, thiamine, and folate. They also contain fiber, essential for the health of the gut. This legume helps lower the bad cholesterol due to low fat content.

- Nuts are legumes that contain high fat content, proteins, carbs, fiber, vitamin E, magnesium, phosphorus, copper, manganese, and selenium. They have been shown to improve gut health and help reduce metabolic syndrome and coronary heart disease.

- Avocados are rich in the healthy monounsaturated fats and are packed with nutrients and vitamins like vitamins C, E, K, and B1 to B6 plus riboflavin, niacin, folic acid, potassium, magnesium, lutein, and beta-carotene. They help you become full and satiated to reduce intake of food. Avocados may help reduce damage to your eyes, support bone health, promote skin health, and may also boost the immune system.

- Seafood and fish are rich in proteins, vitamin D, zinc, iodine, iron, and omega-3 fatty acids. Benefits include improving cell growth, boosting the immune system, lowering heart diseases, and improving brain function. Salmon and fish in general, are easier to digest due to their softer flesh compared to red meat and poultry.

Takeaways from Chapter 7

- Intermittent fasting may reverse type 2 diabetes. But it is important to consult your physician before starting this program to ensure the medication you take matches your new lifestyle.

- Intermittent fasting may help improve the well-being of patients with multiple sclerosis, which affects about 400,000 Americans.

- People with stomach aches can benefit from intermittent fasting as it has been shown to relieve pain.

- Intermittent fasting can help improve brain function including boosting of memory.

- Fasting helps with reducing the speed of aging.

- Heart health is extremely important. Intermittent fasting has been demonstrated to improve heart health by LDL cholesterol. Added benefits include the lowering of blood sugar levels and high blood pressure.

- Intermittent fasting helps with fighting inflammation in the body. This aids the body to avoid certain chronic illnesses such as rheumatoid arthritis and heart disease.

Takeaways from Chapter 8

- Some people battle to lose weight with intermittent fasting 16/8. There are several possible reasons, including:
    - Consuming excessive amounts of carbohydrates.
    - Eating more protein than your body needs.
    - You may experience leptin-resistance and have your appetite always on. Test it if you suspect this may be the issue.
    - Doing too little or excessive physical activity may cause you to not lose weight.
    - Perhaps you aren't sleeping enough.
    - Stress.

- Failure to adapt to intermittent fasting 16/8.
- Drinking alcohol that contains too many carbohydrates.

- Intermittent fasting 16/8 does not cause hair loss.

- Gastritis is caused mainly by bacteria, not intermittent fasting 16/8.

- Most diet plans can reduce both fat mass and fat-free mass. However, intermittent fasting reduces less fat-free mass than other diet plans such as calorie-restricted diets.

- While intermittent fasting, you may have bad breath. This is a sign that your fast is working. The best antidote to bad breath is improved oral hygiene.

- Intermittent fasting by itself does not cause headaches. It is the response to withdrawal of treats like pizzas, chocolate bars, and so on that stresses the body and causes headaches. However, such headaches soon subside.

- Diarrhea can occur during intermittent

fasting. The gut is cleaning itself of toxic material and this is a good thing if not prolonged. If you are concerned about non-stop diarrhea, you may be having an infection or taking medications that cause bacterial imbalance in the stomach.

- You can use intermittent fasting to lose weight even if you have type 2 diabetes. Ensure you consult your medical practitioner before you do so.

Now you have all the information you need to begin losing weight and keep it off permanently by using intermittent fasting 16/8. It's time to get the ball rolling. Most people dilly dally when the time to act arrives. I'm sure you aren't one of them. Let me leave you with a few words of wisdom from Dr. John Tibane, (2017) pastor and author of *Master Your Thought...Transform Your Life*:

"Starting is a proven cure for procrastination." And finally, "Rather deprive your body of sugar and enjoy the sweetness of life than overload your body with sugar and suffer the bitterness of disease."

References

Azevedo, F. R. de, Ikeoka, D., & Caramelli, B. (2013, March 31). Effects of intermittent fasting on metabolism in men. Retrieved from https://www.sciencedirect.com/science/article/pii/S0104423013000213

Berry, S., Valdes, A., Davies, R., Delahanty, L., Drew, D., Chan, A. T., … Spector, T. (2019). Predicting Personal Metabolic Responses to Food Using Multi-omics Machine Learning in over 1000 Twins and Singletons from the UK and US: The PREDICT I Study (OR31-01-19). *Current Developments in Nutrition*, *3*(Supplement_1). doi: 10.1093/cdn/nzz037.or31-01-19

Cardiovascular diseases in Western Pacific. (n.d.). Retrieved from https://www.who.int/westernpacific/health-topics/cardiovascular-diseases

Carter, S., Clifton, P. M., & Keogh, J. B. (2018).

Effect of Intermittent Compared With Continuous Energy Restricted Diet on Glycemic Control in Patients With Type 2 Diabetes. *JAMA Network Open*, *1*(3). doi: 10.1001/jamanetworkopen.2018.0756

Catenacci, V. A., Pan, Z., Ostendorf, D., Brannon, S., Gozansky, W. S., Mattson, M. P., ... Donahoo, W. T. (2016). A randomized pilot study comparing zero-calorie alternate-day fasting to daily caloric restriction in adults with obesity. *Obesity*, *24*(9), 1874–1883. doi: 10.1002/oby.21581

FastStats - Leading Causes of Death. (2017, March 17). Retrieved from https://www.cdc.gov/nchs/fastats/leading-causes-of-death.htm

Fitzgerald, K. C., Vizthum, D., Henry-Barron, B., Schweitzer, A., Cassard, S. D., Kossoff, E., ... Mowry, E. M. (2018). Effect of intermittent vs. daily calorie restriction on changes in weight and patient-reported outcomes in people with multiple sclerosis. *Multiple Sclerosis and Related Disorders*, *23*, 33–39. doi: 10.1016/j.msard.2018.05.002

Fothergill, E., Guo, J., Howard, L., Kerns, J. C., Knuth, N. D., Brychta, R., ... Hall, K. D. (2016). Persistent metabolic adaptation 6 years after "The Biggest Loser" competition. *Obesity*, *24*(8), 1612–1619. doi: 10.1002/oby.21538

Fromentin, C., Tome, D., Nau, F., Flet, L., Luengo, C., Azzout-Marniche, D., ... Gaudichon, C. (2012). Dietary Proteins Contribute Little to Glucose Production, Even Under Optimal Gluconeogenic Conditions in Healthy Humans. *Diabetes*, *62*(5), 1435–1442. doi: 10.2337/db12-1208

Fung, J., & Moore, J. (2016). *The complete guide to fasting: heal your body through intermittent, alternate-day, and extended fasting.*

Fung, J., Fung, J., & Fung, J. (2019, September 26). Dr. Jason Fung: Does fasting burn muscle?

Retrieved from
https://www.dietdoctor.com/does-fasting-burn-muscle

Gabel, K., Hoddy, K. K., Haggerty, N., Song, J., Kroeger, C. M., Trepanowski, J. F., ... Varady, K. A. (2018). Effects of 8-hour time restricted feeding on body weight and metabolic disease risk factors in obese adults: A pilot study. *Nutrition and Healthy Aging*, *4*(4), 345–353. doi: 10.3233/nha-170036

Glick, D., Barth, S., & Macleod, K. F. (2010). Autophagy: cellular and molecular mechanisms. *The Journal of Pathology*, *221*(1), 3–12. doi: 10.1002/path.2697

Guo, E. L., & Katta, R. (2017). Diet and hair loss: effects of nutrient deficiency and supplement use. *Dermatology Practical & Conceptual*, 1–10. doi: 10.5826/dpc.0701a01

Habib, G., Badarny, S., Khreish, M., Khazin, F.,

Shehadeh, V., Hakim, G., & Artul, S. (2014). The Impact of Ramadan Fast on Patients With Gout. *JCR: Journal of Clinical Rheumatology, 20*(7), 353–356. doi: 10.1097/rhu.0000000000000172

Hair Regrowth & Intermittent Fasting: Could This Help? (2020, January 15). Retrieved from https://www.hshairclinic.co.uk/news/will-intermittent-fasting-really-cause-my-hair-to-regrow/

Hjorth, M. F., Astrup, A., Zohar, Y., Urban, L. E., Sayer, R. D., Patterson, B. W., ... Hill, J. O. (2018). Personalized nutrition: pretreatment glucose metabolism determines individual long-term weight loss responsiveness in individuals with obesity on low-carbohydrate versus low-fat diet. *International Journal of Obesity, 43*(10), 2037–2044. doi: 10.1038/s41366-018-0298-4

How to Stop Intermittent Fasting Headaches. (2020, January 29). Retrieved from https://dofasting.com/blog/intermittent-fasting-headache/

Huda. (2019, January 19). Do Muslim Children Fast During Ramadan? Retrieved from https://www.learnreligions.com/children-and-fasting-during-ramadan-2004614

Hypoglycaemia. (n.d.). Retrieved from https://www.migrainetrust.org/about-migraine/trigger-factors/hypoglycaemia/

IDF Diabetes Atlas 9th edition 2019. (n.d.). Retrieved from https://www.diabetesatlas.org/

Johnson, J. B., Summer, W., Cutler, R. G., Martin, B., Hyun, D.-H., Dixit, V. D., ... Mattson, M. P. (2007). Alternate day calorie restriction improves clinical findings and reduces markers of oxidative stress and inflammation in overweight adults with moderate asthma. *Free Radical Biology and Medicine, 42*(5), 665–674. doi: 10.1016/j.freeradbiomed.2006.12.005

Klok, M. D., Jakobsdottir, S., & Drent, M. L. (2007). The role of leptin and ghrelin in the regulation of food intake and body weight in humans: a review. *Obesity Reviews*, *8*(1), 21–34. doi: 10.1111/j.1467-789x.2006.00270.x

Knuth, N. D., Johannsen, D. L., Tamboli, R. A., Marks-Shulman, P. A., Huizenga, R., Chen, K. Y., … Hall, K. D. (2014). Metabolic adaptation following massive weight loss is related to the degree of energy imbalance and changes in circulating leptin. *Obesity*. doi: 10.1002/oby.20900

Land, S. (2018). *Metabolic Autophagy: Practice Intermittent Fasting and Resistance Training to Build Muscle and Promote Longevity*. Independently Published.

Lanham-New, S. A. (2009). *Introduction to Human Nutrition* (Second). Wiley-Blackwell.

Livingston, G. (2015). *Never binge again: reprogram yourself to think like a permanently thin person, stop overeating and binge eating and stick to the food plan of your choice!* North Charleston, SC: CreateSpace Independent Publishing Platform.

Maltz, M. (1960). *Psycho-cybernetic principles: a new way to get more living out of life.* Chatsworth, CA: Wilshire Book Co.

Mattson, M. P., Longo, V. D., & Harvie, M. (2017). Impact of intermittent fasting on health and disease processes. *Ageing Research Reviews, 39,* 46–58. doi: 10.1016/j.arr.2016.10.005

Nedeltcheva, A. V., Kilkus, J. M., Imperial, J., Schoeller, D. A., & Penev, P. D. (2010). Insufficient Sleep Undermines Dietary Efforts to Reduce Adiposity. *Annals of Internal Medicine, 153*(7), 435. doi: 10.7326/0003-4819-153-7-201010050-00006

Qi, L. (2014). Personalized nutrition and obesity. *Annals of Medicine, 46*(5), 247–252. doi: 10.3109/07853890.2014.891802

Reporter, D. M. (2013, September 16). Diet starts today... and ends on Friday: How we quickly slip back into bad eating habits within a few days. Retrieved from https://www.dailymail.co.uk/news/article-2421737/Diet-starts-today--ends-Friday-How-quickly-slip-bad-eating-habits-days.html

Rossi, C. (2019, February 16). The Reason Intermittent Fasting Is Giving You Bad Breath. Retrieved from https://www.popsugar.com.au/fitness/How-Stop-Bad-Breath-When-Dieting-Fasting-44060243

SHELTON, H. (1978). *Science And Fine Art Of Fasting*.

Shin, B. K., Kang, S., Kim, D. S., & Park, S. (2018). Intermittent fasting protects against the deterioration of cognitive function, energy metabolism and dyslipidemia in Alzheimer's disease-induced estrogen deficient rats. *Experimental Biology and Medicine, 243*(4), 334–343. doi: 10.1177/1535370217751610

Tibane, J. (2007). *Master Your Thoughts...Transform Your Life: thinking styles and practices to achieve ultimate success.* Struik Inspirational, Tiger Valley.

The Science. (2020, January 6). Retrieved from https://thefastingmethod.com/the-science/

Tokede, O. A., Onabanjo, T. A., Yansane, A., Gaziano, J. M., & Djoussé, L. (2015). Soya products and serum lipids: a meta-analysis of randomised controlled trials. *British Journal of Nutrition, 114*(6), 831–843. doi: 10.1017/s0007114515002603

Toro-Martín, J. D., Arsenault, B., Després, J.-P., & Vohl, M.-C. (2017). Precision Nutrition: A Review of Personalized Nutritional Approaches for the Prevention and Management of Metabolic Syndrome. *Nutrients*, *9*(8), 913. doi: 10.3390/nu9080913

Varady, K. A., Bhutani, S., Church, E. C., & Klempel, M. C. (2009). Short-term modified alternate-day fasting: a novel dietary strategy for weight loss and cardioprotection in obese adults. *The American Journal of Clinical Nutrition*, *90*(5), 1138–1143. doi: 10.3945/ajcn.2009.28380

Williams, R.J. (1998). *Biochemical Individuality : The Basis for the Genetotrophic Concept*. NTC Contemporary.

Yu, C. W. and W. (2019, March 8). Gastritis: Causes, Diagnosis, and Treatment. Retrieved from https://www.healthline.com/health/gastritis

Zeevi, D., Korem, T., Zmora, N., Israeli, D., Rothschild, D., Weinberger, A., ... Segal, E. (2015). Personalized Nutrition by Prediction of Glycemic Responses. *Cell*, *163*(5), 1079–1094. doi: 10.1016/j.cell.2015.11.001

Printed in Great Britain
by Amazon